Pharmacology Pulse: 2800 Rapidfire One-Liners for NEET PG

Copyright Page

Title: NEET PG Pulse: Pharmacology 2800 MCQs Topic-wise with Explanations

Author: Dr (Major) Debasish Das

Publisher: NEET PG Pulse

Edition: First Edition, 2024

ISBN: 978-93-342-9198-8

Disclaimer:
The content of this book is intended for educational purposes only. While every effort has been made to ensure the accuracy of the material, the author and publisher shall not be held responsible for any consequences arising from the use of this book in medical decision-making. Always consult updated guidelines and clinical judgment.
Always consult updated guidelines and clinical judgment.

Dedication

To every medical student who has fought sleepless nights and endless stress with relentless passion.

Preface

This book is designed to help NEET PG aspirants master Pharmacology through focused, topic-wise MCQs with concise explanations. It combines past-year patterns, updated clinical insights, and exam-aligned one-liners across all essential pharmacology domains. With over 2800 MCQs classified into 14 structured chapters, this resource ensures a complete and engaging preparation strategy.

Whether you're revising late into the night or brushing up during rotations, this book will guide you question by question—towards conceptual clarity and confident performance.

How to Use This Book

This book is structured to give you the **fastest possible revision of Pharmacology**—ideal for NEET PG and other competitive exams.

- Topics are arranged in **clearly separated sections** for focused study.
- Includes the **most frequently asked questions** and **PYQs** from the last 10 years.
- Designed to be completed in **just 7 days**—perfect for **busy interns, residents, or working doctors** who don't have time for lengthy coaching or textbooks.

Use it as your **last-mile revision tool** to boost recall and confidence right before the exam.

About the Author

Dr (Major) Debasish Das, MBBS (Trivandrum), MD (Army Hospital R&R, New Delhi), is a Consultant Anesthesiologist and Intensivist at Assam Cancer Care Foundation. With years of academic and clinical excellence, Dr. Das has trained countless students for NEET PG and licensing exams. His focused approach blends concise medical content with real-world applicability—making complex topics easy, memorable, and exam-ready.

He is also the creator of the **Sniper NEET PG Vol. 1: PSM, Pathology & Microbiology** – 10 Years Recall + Ultrafast Revision MCQs - built to deliver precision, affordability, and power-packed content for the modern aspirant.

General Pharmacology

Q1. Bioavailability of IV drugs?
100%
IV drugs bypass first-pass metabolism.

Q2. First-pass metabolism occurs in?
Liver
Oral drugs are metabolized here before systemic circulation.

Q3. Drug with zero-order kinetics?
Phenytoin
Fixed amount eliminated per unit time (not proportion).

Q4. Volume of distribution depends on?
Lipid solubility and protein binding
Highly lipid-soluble drugs have large Vd.

Q5. Therapeutic index is calculated as?
TD50 / ED50
Higher TI = safer drug.

Q6. Loading dose depends on?
Volume of distribution
Achieves target plasma concentration rapidly.

Q7. Maintenance dose depends on?
Clearance and bioavailability
Keeps drug levels steady.

Q8. Prodrug example?
Enalapril
Converted to active form (enalaprilat) in liver.

Q9. First-order kinetics means?
Constant fraction of drug eliminated per unit time
Most drugs follow this.

Q10. Zero-order drugs?
Phenytoin, Ethanol, Aspirin (at high doses)
Elimination is saturable.

Q11. Bioavailability of oral propranolol?
Low
Due to extensive first-pass metabolism.

Q12. Drug with high plasma protein binding?
Warfarin
>90% protein-bound, narrow therapeutic index.

Q13. Half-life formula?
$0.693 \times Vd / Clearance$
Time taken for plasma concentration to halve.

Q14. Drug elimination mainly via kidneys?
Aminoglycosides
Dose adjustment needed in renal impairment.

Q15. Drug clearance depends on?
Renal/hepatic function and drug metabolism
Determines maintenance dose.

Q16. Drug with low Vd likely stays in?
Plasma
Hydrophilic and highly protein-bound.

Q17. Phase I reactions include?
Oxidation, reduction, hydrolysis
Introduces polar groups.

Q18. Phase II reactions?
Conjugation (glucuronidation, acetylation, etc.)
Makes drug water-soluble.

Q19. Drug with poor oral bioavailability?
Nitroglycerin
Rapidly metabolized by liver.

Q20. CYP450 enzyme inducer?
Rifampin
Increases metabolism of other drugs.

Q21. CYP450 inhibitor?
Erythromycin
Decreases metabolism → drug toxicity risk.

Q22. Drug acting via G-protein coupled receptor?
Adrenaline
Acts on adrenergic receptors.

Q23. Drug with narrow therapeutic index?
Digoxin
Requires therapeutic drug monitoring.

Q24. First-order drug accumulation leads to?
Steady state
Achieved after ~4–5 half-lives.

Q25. Drug displacement from albumin increases?
Free (active) drug level
Increases toxicity risk.

Q26. Acidic drugs bind to?
Albumin
Basic drugs bind to alpha-1 glycoprotein.

Q27. pKa of a drug indicates?
pH at which 50% is ionized
Important for absorption prediction.

Q28. Ion trapping occurs where?
In renal tubules
Weak acids excreted more in alkaline urine.

Q29. Drug efficacy is defined as?
Maximal response a drug can produce
Different from potency.

Q30. Drug potency refers to?
Dose required to produce effect
More potent = lower dose needed.

Q31. Drug with highest first-pass metabolism?
Propranolol
Extensive hepatic metabolism before entering systemic circulation.

Q32. Drug best absorbed in acidic pH?
Aspirin
It is a weak acid, absorbed in stomach.

Q33. Bioavailability of sublingual route?
High
Bypasses first-pass metabolism.

Q34. Drug best given by transdermal route?
Nitroglycerin
Provides slow, sustained absorption.

Q35. Intramuscular absorption is faster with?
Aqueous solutions
Oily injections absorb slower.

Q36. Route of administration with fastest action?
IV bolus
Immediate entry into circulation.

Q37. Inhalational agents show fast action due to?
Large surface area and rich blood supply
Also avoids hepatic metabolism.

Q38. Depot preparations release drug?
Slowly over time
IM oily injections (e.g., penicillin G benzathine).

Q39. Subcutaneous route used for?
Insulin, heparin
Suitable for self-administration.

Q40. Volume of distribution of digoxin?
Large
Enters extensively into tissues.

Q41. Drug interaction increases when two drugs?
Compete for same plasma protein binding
Example: warfarin and sulfonamides.

Q42. Drugs eliminated by zero-order kinetics?
Phenytoin, Ethanol, Aspirin (high doses)
Fixed amount eliminated per time.

Q43. Enterohepatic circulation prolongs?
Drug half-life
e.g., oral contraceptives, chloramphenicol.

Q44. pH of urine affects excretion of?
Weak acids/bases
Alkaline urine → acidic drug excretion ↑.

Q45. Steady state is achieved after?
4–5 half-lives
Applies to continuous drug dosing.

Q46. Area under the curve (AUC) represents?
Total drug exposure
Used in bioavailability & bioequivalence.

Q47. Bioequivalence means?
Similar rate and extent of absorption
Same AUC, Cmax, Tmax.

Q48. Drug with active metabolite?
Diazepam
Converted to desmethyldiazepam.

Q49. Drug not requiring metabolism?
Lithium
Excreted unchanged in urine.

Q50. Drug given via rectal route avoids?
Partial first-pass metabolism
Especially in lower rectum absorption.

Q51. Highly lipid-soluble drug characteristic?
Large Vd
Easily crosses membranes.

Q52. What is clearance?
Volume of plasma cleared of drug per unit time
CL = Rate of elimination / Plasma conc.

Q53. Loading dose = ?
(Target concentration × Vd) / Bioavailability
Used for immediate effect.

Q54. Drug TDM is needed for?
Narrow therapeutic index drugs
Eg. digoxin, lithium, aminoglycosides.

Q55. Drug with low oral bioavailability?
Dobutamine
Rapidly destroyed in GIT or liver.

Q56. Lipophilic drugs stored in?
Fat tissue
Prolonged action possible.

Q57. Plasma concentration-time curve shows?
Cmax, Tmax, AUC
Helps calculate half-life and bioavailability.

Q58. Therapeutic window is?
Range between minimum effective and toxic dose
Determines safe dosing range.

Q59. Drug efficacy curve shifts?
Vertically
Indicates how well drug works.

Q60. Potency curve shifts?
Horizontally
Indicates required dose for effect.

Q61. Drug interaction by enzyme induction leads to?
Decreased plasma levels of co-administered drug
Inducers like rifampin speed up metabolism.

Q62. Drug interaction by enzyme inhibition leads to?
Increased drug toxicity
Example: erythromycin with theophylline.

Q63. First-order kinetics graph is?
Log-linear
Shows exponential decline.

Q64. Drug that does not follow first-pass effect?
Sublingual nitroglycerin
Directly enters systemic circulation.

Q65. Example of a prodrug activated in liver?
Enalapril → Enalaprilat
Needs metabolic conversion.

Q66. Which property affects half-life?
Volume of distribution and clearance
$t½ = 0.693 \times Vd / CL$

Q67. Ionized form of drug is?
Less lipid-soluble
Poorly absorbed across membranes.

Q68. Basic drugs are absorbed best at?
Alkaline pH
Non-ionized form predominates.

Q69. Acidic drugs absorbed best at?
Acidic pH
e.g., Aspirin in stomach.

Q70. Competitive antagonism shifts dose-response curve?
Rightward
Maximal response remains unchanged.

Q71. Non-competitive antagonism effect?
Lowers maximum response
Binds irreversibly or allosterically.

Q72. Agonist + antagonist together leads to?
Partial effect
Depends on their relative affinities.

Q73. Potency comparison uses?
EC50 values
Lower EC50 = more potent.

Q74. Drug with short half-life needs?
Frequent dosing
To maintain steady plasma levels.

Q75. Mechanism of drug resistance?
Enzyme modification, efflux pumps, receptor alteration
Common in antimicrobials.

Q76. Phase 1 clinical trial focuses on?
Safety and pharmacokinetics
Done on healthy volunteers.

Q77. Phase 2 clinical trial goal?
Efficacy and dose range
Small group of patients.

Q78. Phase 3 trial evaluates?
Comparison with standard therapy
Large-scale patient groups.

Q79. Phase 4 trial is done for?
Post-marketing surveillance
Detects long-term side effects.

Q80. Orphan drug is used for?
Rare diseases
Not profitable for large-scale production.

Q81. Drug schedule with highest abuse potential?
Schedule I (e.g., LSD)
No accepted medical use.

Q82. Drug schedule with medical use but abuse risk?
Schedule II (e.g., morphine)
Strict regulation.

Q83. Drug allergy is classified as?
Type I–IV hypersensitivity
Common in penicillin.

Q84. Tachyphylaxis refers to?
Rapid tolerance
Seen with nitrates, ephedrine.

Q85. Idiosyncratic reaction is?
Unpredictable and genetic
e.g., G6PD deficiency and sulfa drugs.

Q86. Teratogenicity means?
Drug-induced fetal abnormalities
e.g., thalidomide, isotretinoin.

Q87. Category X drug in pregnancy?
Contraindicated
Risk outweighs benefit.

Q88. Which drugs cross placenta easily?
Lipid-soluble, low MW drugs
e.g., warfarin.

Q89. Which drugs are excreted in breast milk?
Weak bases and lipophilic drugs
e.g., tetracycline, phenobarbital.

Q90. Elderly have decreased?
Renal clearance
Dose adjustment often needed.

Q91. Best route for drugs with high first-pass metabolism?
Sublingual or transdermal
Avoids hepatic inactivation.

Q92. What is the inverse agonist?
Drug that produces opposite effect of agonist
e.g., propranolol at β-receptors.

Q93. Example of a partial agonist?
Buprenorphine
Less efficacy than full agonist.

Q94. Drug synergism means?
Combined effect > sum of individual effects
Example: Sulfonamide + Trimethoprim.

Q95. Potency comparison uses?
EC50 value
Lower EC50 = more potent.

Q96. Therapeutic index of warfarin?
Narrow
Requires close INR monitoring.

Q97. Drug with high first-pass effect?
Labetalol
Requires larger oral dose.

Q98. Clearance of drug increases with?
Enzyme induction
Rifampin, phenytoin induce CYP450.

Q99. Most common Phase I reaction?
Oxidation
Makes drug more polar.

Q100. Phase II reactions form?
Conjugated metabolites
Glucuronidation, sulfation, etc.

Q101. Drug microsomal enzymes found in?
Liver smooth endoplasmic reticulum
Involved in metabolism.

Q102. Microsomal enzyme inducers?
Rifampin, phenobarbital
Increase drug metabolism.

Q103. Microsomal enzyme inhibitors?
Cimetidine, ketoconazole
May increase toxicity of other drugs.

Q104. Non-microsomal metabolism site?
Plasma, cytosol
e.g., acetylation, hydrolysis.

Q105. Non-microsomal enzymes?
Pseudocholinesterase
Breaks down succinylcholine.

Q106. Drug acetylation polymorphism affects?
Isoniazid metabolism
Slow acetylators → more side effects.

Q107. Drug with significant genetic polymorphism?
Isoniazid
Acetylation rate differs among individuals.

Q108. Drug metabolism in neonates is?
Slower
Immature liver enzymes.

Q109. Geriatric patients show?
↓ Renal clearance
Risk of accumulation & toxicity.

Q110. Loading dose example drug?
Digoxin
Given to rapidly achieve effect.

Q111. Maintenance dose depends on?
Clearance & bioavailability
Keeps plasma levels steady.

Q112. Ionization affects?
Drug absorption
Non-ionized = better absorbed.

Q113. Lipid solubility affects?
Distribution
Lipid-soluble = high Vd.

Q114. Highly ionized drugs are?
Poorly absorbed
Cannot cross membranes easily.

Q115. Highly plasma protein-bound drug?
Warfarin
Lowers free (active) concentration.

Q116. Drug with active metabolites?
Diazepam
Prolonged duration of action.

Q117. Enterohepatic circulation prolongs action of?
Estrogens, rifampin
Reabsorbed from intestine.

Q118. Clearance is measured in?
mL/min
Represents plasma cleared per time.

Q119. Hepatic clearance depends on?
Liver enzyme activity
Influenced by inhibitors/inducers.

Q120. Renal clearance is affected by?
GFR, secretion, reabsorption
Used for dose adjustment in renal failure.

Q121. Dose-response curve shifts right with?
Competitive antagonist
Requires more agonist to achieve same effect.

Q122. Ceiling effect is seen with?
Partial agonists
Max response is lower than full agonists.

Q123. Drug interaction via absorption change?
Antacids + tetracycline
Chelation reduces absorption.

Q124. Receptor upregulation occurs after?
Prolonged antagonist use
Increases receptor sensitivity.

Q125. Downregulation occurs after?
Chronic agonist exposure
Receptor desensitization.

Q126. EC50 means?
Drug concentration at 50% of max effect
Measure of potency.

Q127. LD50 is used for?
Estimating drug toxicity
Dose causing death in 50% of animals.

Q128. Drug with narrow safety margin?
Theophylline
Requires close monitoring.

Q129. High lipid solubility leads to?
High Vd
Drug stays in tissues.

Q130. Drug with low bioavailability orally?
Lidocaine
Extensive hepatic metabolism.

Q131. Glucuronidation is absent in?
Neonates
Risk of gray baby syndrome (chloramphenicol).

Q132. Example of drug interaction via protein displacement?
Warfarin + sulfonamides
Increases free warfarin → bleeding.

Q133. Enzyme induction develops slowly because?
Needs protein synthesis
Takes a few days to manifest.

Q134. Drug example with enzyme inhibition?
Cimetidine
Inhibits CYP450 → prolongs action of other drugs.

Q135. Which route has no absorption phase?
IV route
Direct to bloodstream.

Q136. Drug storage in fat leads to?
Slow elimination
Example: thiopental.

Q137. Therapeutic drug monitoring used for?
Lithium
Narrow therapeutic window.

Q138. Enteral route includes?
Oral, sublingual, rectal
All use GI tract.

Q139. Parenteral route example?
IM injection
Avoids first-pass metabolism.

Q140. Glomerular filtration clears?
Free, unbound drugs
Protein-bound drugs are not filtered.

Q141. Active tubular secretion site?
Proximal tubule
For organic acids/bases.

Q142. Tubular reabsorption depends on?
Urine pH and drug pKa
Affects ionization.

Q143. Acidic drug excretion ↑ in?
Alkaline urine
Done in salicylate poisoning.

Q144. Basic drug excretion ↑ in?
Acidic urine
Ion trapping principle.

Q145. Drug effect correlates with?
Free plasma concentration
Not total level.

Q146. Which drug follows perfusion-limited distribution?
Lipid-soluble drugs
Quickly enter tissues.

Q147. Protein-limited distribution seen in?
Hydrophilic drugs
Limited membrane crossing.

Q148. Neonatal drug metabolism is?
Decreased
Enzyme systems are immature.

Q149. Renal function is assessed by?
Creatinine clearance
Used to adjust dosing.

Q150. Drug bound to albumin is?
Inactive
Only free drug is pharmacologically active.

Q151. Steady state is achieved faster with?
Shorter half-life
4–5 half-lives needed for steady state.

Q152. Bioavailability of rectal route?
Intermediate
Bypasses partial first-pass metabolism.

Q153. Most rapid absorption (oral)?
Sublingual
Bypasses liver and enters systemic circulation directly.

Q154. Drug monitoring needed for?
Carbamazepine
Narrow therapeutic range.

Q155. Drug excreted unchanged in urine?
Aminoglycosides
Nephrotoxic and renally cleared.

Q156. Long acting benzodiazepine?
Diazepam
Forms active metabolites.

Q157. Dose adjustment in renal failure?
Required for renally excreted drugs
E.g., digoxin, aminoglycosides.

Q158. Clearance is zero at?
Equilibrium
When drug input = output.

Q159. Bioequivalence indicates?
Same AUC, Cmax, Tmax
Similar efficacy and safety.

Q160. Non-ionized form of drug?
Lipid soluble
Easily crosses membranes.

Q161. Maximum drug response =
Efficacy
Not related to potency.

Q162. Enzyme inducer effect on warfarin?
↓ Effect
Increased metabolism → INR drops.

Q163. Enzyme inhibitor effect on warfarin?
↑ Effect
Risk of bleeding.

Q164. Most significant site for drug excretion?
Kidneys
Renal failure = dose adjustment.

Q165. Drug metabolized by acetylation?
Isoniazid
Rate differs by genetic type.

Q166. Gray baby syndrome due to?
Chloramphenicol
Immature glucuronidation in neonates.

Q167. Volume of distribution of heparin?
Low
Confined to plasma.

Q168. Ion trapping used for?
Enhancing drug excretion
e.g., salicylate poisoning.

Q169. Non-competitive antagonist binds?
Irreversibly
Reduces maximum response.

Q170. Full agonist produces?
Maximum possible effect
e.g., morphine at μ-opioid receptor.

Q171. Partial agonist effect?
Submaximal response
Even at full receptor occupancy.

Q172. Bioavailability of IM injection?
High but variable
Depends on perfusion and formulation.

Q173. Factors increasing drug clearance?
Enzyme induction, increased renal perfusion
Results in reduced drug levels.

Q174. Weak bases are excreted more in?
Acidic urine
e.g., amphetamines.

Q175. Weak acids excreted more in?
Alkaline urine
Used in aspirin overdose.

Q176. pKa = pH means drug is?
50% ionized
Point of maximal buffering.

Q177. Placenta favors passage of?
Lipid-soluble, non-ionized drugs
Crosses easily.

Q178. Drug reabsorption occurs in?
Renal tubules
Passive for lipid-soluble drugs.

Q179. Drug secretion occurs in?
Proximal tubule
Via active transport.

Q180. Phase I metabolism leads to?
Activation, inactivation, or toxicity
Often creates reactive intermediates.

Q181. Most important organ for drug metabolism?
Liver
Contains microsomal enzymes (CYP450).

Q182. Drug given as loading dose?
Digoxin
Rapidly achieves therapeutic levels.

Q183. Target concentration concept is used for?
Maintenance dose calculation
Ensures steady drug level.

Q184. IV bolus results in?
Immediate peak concentration
No absorption delay.

Q185. Effect of protein binding on half-life?
Increases
Delays elimination of free drug.

Q186. Lipid-soluble drugs stored in?
Fat tissues
Delays elimination.

Q187. Hydrophilic drugs remain in?
Plasma and interstitial fluid
Low volume of distribution.

Q188. Highly polar drugs excreted via?
Kidney
Cannot cross membranes easily.

Q189. Drug with negligible first-pass effect?
Isosorbide dinitrate (sublingual)
Avoids liver.

Q190. Log dose-response curve shape?
Sigmoid
Standard pharmacologic graph.

Q191. Competitive inhibition reversibility?
Reversible
Can be overcome by high agonist dose.

Q192. Receptor reserve means?
Spare receptors
Full response with less than full occupancy.

Q193. Latent period relates to?
Onset of drug action
Affected by absorption rate.

Q194. Area under curve (AUC) in graph shows?
Total drug exposure
Reflects bioavailability.

Q195. Therapeutic range is between?
MEC and MTC
Minimum effective and toxic concentrations.

Q196. Drug efficacy depends on?
Intrinsic activity
Not affected by affinity or EC50.

Q197. EC50 is low for?
Highly potent drugs
Requires small dose.

Q198. Drug bioavailability is affected by?

First-pass metabolism, formulation, solubility
Oral vs IV differs greatly.

Q199. Acidification of urine promotes excretion of?

Weak bases
Example: amphetamine.

Q200. Alkalinization of urine promotes excretion of?

Weak acids
Used in aspirin (salicylate) overdose.

Autonomic Nervous System Pharmacology

Q1. Neurotransmitter at all autonomic ganglia?
Acetylcholine
Acts on nicotinic receptors.

Q2. Parasympathetic postganglionic neurotransmitter?
Acetylcholine
Acts on muscarinic receptors.

Q3. Sympathetic postganglionic neurotransmitter?
Norepinephrine
Except sweat glands (ACh).

Q4. Receptor at neuromuscular junction?
Nicotinic (Nm)
Found in skeletal muscle.

Q5. Muscarinic receptors are?
G-protein coupled
M1, M2, M3 types.

Q6. Nicotinic receptors are?
Ligand-gated ion channels
Found in ganglia and NMJ.

Q7. M2 receptors are located in?
Heart
Cause bradycardia via vagus.

Q8. M3 receptor stimulation causes?
Smooth muscle contraction & glandular secretion
Also causes miosis.

Q9. β1 receptors are located in?
Heart and juxtaglomerular cells
Increase HR, contractility, renin.

Q10. β2 receptor stimulation leads to?
Bronchodilation
Also causes vasodilation in skeletal muscle.

Q11. α1 receptor activation causes?

Vasoconstriction

Used in nasal decongestants.

Q12. α2 receptor location and effect?

Presynaptic terminals

Inhibits norepinephrine release.

Q13. Dopamine at low dose acts on?

D1 receptors

Causes renal vasodilation.

Q14. Isoproterenol is selective for?

β1 and β2 receptors

Non-selective β agonist.

Q15. Phenylephrine acts on?

α1 receptors

Used for hypotension and nasal congestion.

Q16. Clonidine acts on?

α2 receptors (central)

Lowers BP by reducing sympathetic outflow.

Q17. Salbutamol is selective for?

β2 receptors

Used in bronchial asthma.

Q18. Dobutamine mainly acts on?

β1 receptors

Increases cardiac output in heart failure.

Q19. Effect of atropine on heart?

Tachycardia

Blocks vagal M2 receptors.

Q20. Cholinergic crisis treated with?

Atropine

Antidote for organophosphate poisoning.

Q21. Neostigmine mechanism?

Acetylcholinesterase inhibitor

Increases ACh at synapse.

Q22. Physostigmine vs neostigmine?
Physostigmine crosses BBB
Used in atropine overdose.

Q23. Edrophonium use?
Diagnosis of myasthenia gravis
Short-acting AChE inhibitor.

Q24. Myasthenia treatment drug?
Pyridostigmine
Long-acting AChE inhibitor.

Q25. Cholinergic side effects?
SLUDGE: Salivation, Lacrimation, Urination, Defecation, GI upset, Emesis
Muscarinic overactivity.

Q26. Anticholinergic side effects?
Dry mouth, blurred vision, tachycardia, urinary retention
Seen with atropine, TCAs.

Q27. Reversal of non-depolarizing muscle relaxants?
Neostigmine + Atropine
Atropine prevents bradycardia.

Q28. Succinylcholine is?
Depolarizing neuromuscular blocker
Short-acting, Phase I + II block.

Q29. Non-depolarizing blocker example?
Vecuronium
Competitive antagonist at Nm receptor.

Q30. Succinylcholine side effects?
Hyperkalemia, malignant hyperthermia
Also causes bradycardia.

Q31. Drug of choice for organophosphate poisoning?
Atropine + Pralidoxime
Atropine blocks muscarinic effects, pralidoxime reactivates AChE.

Q32. Pralidoxime is effective only in?
Early stages of OP poisoning
Before enzyme aging occurs.

Q33. Beta-blocker with intrinsic sympathomimetic activity?

Pindolol

Partial agonist, less bradycardia.

Q34. Beta-blocker selective for β1?

Atenolol

Safer in asthmatics.

Q35. Non-selective beta-blocker?

Propranolol

Blocks both β1 and β2 receptors.

Q36. Labetalol blocks?

α1, β1, β2

Used in hypertensive emergencies.

Q37. Beta-blocker used in glaucoma?

Timolol

Reduces aqueous humor production.

Q38. Reserpine mechanism?

Depletes catecholamines from storage vesicles

Causes sedation, depression.

Q39. Drug that inhibits reuptake of norepinephrine?

Cocaine

Also local anesthetic.

Q40. Alpha-1 blocker used in BPH?

Tamsulosin

Selective for prostate smooth muscle.

Q41. Drug causing first dose hypotension?

Prazosin

Start with low dose at bedtime.

Q42. Ganglion blocker example?

Trimethaphan

Obsolete antihypertensive.

Q43. Side effect of α2 agonist (e.g., clonidine)?

Rebound hypertension

On sudden withdrawal.

Q44. Alpha-methyl dopa used in?
Hypertension in pregnancy
Safe and effective.

Q45. Action of epinephrine on BP?
Biphasic: α1 ↑BP, β2 ↓BP
Net effect depends on dose.

Q46. Epinephrine reversal seen with?
α-blockers
Unmasks β2 vasodilation → ↓BP.

Q47. Tyramine causes?
Indirect sympathomimetic action
Can precipitate hypertensive crisis with MAOIs.

Q48. Amphetamines act by?
Releasing stored catecholamines
CNS stimulant.

Q49. Adverse effect of beta-blockers in diabetes?
Masking hypoglycemia
Inhibits tachycardia response.

Q50. Beta-blocker contraindicated in asthma?
Non-selective β-blockers (e.g., propranolol)
Risk of bronchospasm.

Q51. Alpha-1 receptor activation causes?
Vasoconstriction and pupil dilation
Used in nasal decongestants.

Q52. Beta-2 receptor activation causes?
Bronchodilation and uterine relaxation
Salbutamol used in asthma, preterm labor.

Q53. Beta-3 receptor found in?
Adipose tissue
Promotes lipolysis.

Q54. Side effect of β-blockers?
Bradycardia, fatigue, depression, ED
Dose-dependent.

Q55. Pilocarpine used in?
Glaucoma and xerostomia
Muscarinic agonist.

Q56. Muscarinic antagonist for motion sickness?
Scopolamine
CNS-acting anticholinergic.

Q57. Atropine overdose features?
Dry mouth, tachycardia, hyperthermia, delirium
"Hot as hare, dry as bone..."

Q58. Reversal agent for atropine overdose?
Physostigmine
Crosses BBB to reverse CNS effects.

Q59. Bethanechol used in?
Atonic bladder, postoperative ileus
Muscarinic agonist.

Q60. Contraindications to cholinomimetics?
Asthma, peptic ulcer, bradycardia
Risk of worsening symptoms.

Q61. Which cholinomimetic is resistant to AChE?
Bethanechol
Longer duration of action.

Q62. Drug increasing salivation in Sjögren's syndrome?
Pilocarpine
Muscarinic agonist.

Q63. Which drug mimics parasympathetic action?
Muscarine
Found in certain mushrooms.

Q64. Which toxin causes irreversible AChE inhibition?
Organophosphates
Requires pralidoxime + atropine.

Q65. Mydriasis without cycloplegia caused by?
Phenylephrine
$\alpha 1$ agonist, no accommodation paralysis.

Q66. Antidote for organophosphate poisoning?
Pralidoxime
Reactivates AChE if given early.

Q67. Anticholinergic used for Parkinson's?
Benztropine
Reduces tremor and rigidity.

Q68. Drug that causes cycloplegia and mydriasis?
Atropine
Muscarinic blocker.

Q69. Muscarinic blocker used in asthma (inhaled)?
Ipratropium
Bronchodilator with minimal systemic effects.

Q70. CNS side effect of atropine?
Delirium
Especially in elderly.

Q71. Non-depolarizing muscle relaxant with short duration?
Mivacurium
Rapidly hydrolyzed by plasma cholinesterase.

Q72. Depolarizing blocker that causes fasciculations?
Succinylcholine
Phase I block.

Q73. Adverse effect of prolonged succinylcholine?
Malignant hyperthermia
Treat with dantrolene.

Q74. Which receptor mediates detrusor contraction?
M3
Causes urination.

Q75. Which receptor mediates bladder sphincter relaxation?
M3
Parasympathetic effect.

Q76. Drug causing paradoxical bradycardia in low dose?
Atropine
Via central vagal stimulation.

Q77. Which drug increases systolic and diastolic BP and reflex bradycardia?
Norepinephrine
Via α1 and β1 action.

Q78. Drug with β2 > β1 action?
Salmeterol
Long-acting bronchodilator.

Q79. Side effect of β2 agonists?
Tremor
Due to skeletal muscle stimulation.

Q80. Selective α1 blocker for hypertension + BPH?
Doxazosin
Dual benefit.

Q81. Drug that increases BP and HR?
Epinephrine (high dose)
α and β1 stimulation.

Q82. β1 selective blocker with short half-life?
Esmolol
Used IV in acute arrhythmias.

Q83. Antihypertensive acting centrally via α2 receptors?
Clonidine
Decreases sympathetic tone.

Q84. α1 antagonist used in pheochromocytoma?
Phenoxybenzamine
Irreversible blocker.

Q85. Which drug causes reflex tachycardia?
Prazosin
Due to vasodilation and BP drop.

Q86. Vasoconstrictor used in nasal congestion?
Oxymetazoline
α1 agonist.

Q87. Beta-blocker with membrane stabilizing activity?
Propranolol
Not used for anti-arrhythmic effect.

Q88. Sympathetic stimulation increases BP via?
α1 and β1 receptors
Vasoconstriction + ↑ CO.

Q89. Sympathetic effect on eye?
Mydriasis
Radial muscle contraction (α1).

Q90. Parasympathetic effect on eye?
Miosis and accommodation
M3 receptor mediated.

Q91. Adrenergic agonist used to delay premature labor?
Ritodrine
β2 agonist → uterine relaxation.

Q92. Which receptor mediates uterine relaxation?
β2
Smooth muscle relaxation in uterus.

Q93. α2 agonist causing dry mouth & sedation?
Clonidine
Central sympatholytic.

Q94. β-blocker preferred in COPD patients?
Atenolol
β1 selective, spares β2.

Q95. β-blocker causing dyslipidemia?
Propranolol
Increases TG, decreases HDL.

Q96. Sympathetic receptor that inhibits insulin secretion?
α2
Found on pancreatic β-cells.

Q97. Sympathetic receptor that promotes insulin release?
β2
Stimulates insulin via cAMP.

Q98. β-blocker used for migraine prophylaxis?
Propranolol
CNS effects reduce frequency.

Q99. Receptor that increases renin secretion?
β1
Found in juxtaglomerular cells.

Q100. β-blocker with vasodilatory property?
Nebivolol
Releases NO.

Q101. β-blocker used for hypertrophic cardiomyopathy?
Propranolol
Reduces outflow obstruction.

Q102. Non-selective α-blocker?
Phenoxybenzamine
Used preoperatively in pheochromocytoma.

Q103. Short-acting α-blocker for phaeo crisis?
Phentolamine
Reversible α1/α2 blocker.

Q104. α2 agonist side effect?
Sedation, rebound hypertension
Seen with clonidine.

Q105. Muscarinic receptor antagonist used in IBS?
Dicyclomine
Relieves GI spasms.

Q106. Which receptor stimulates salivation?
M3
Parasympathetic effect.

Q107. Ganglion blockers lower BP by?
Blocking sympathetic tone
Obsolete due to side effects.

Q108. Drug causing miosis?
Pilocarpine
Muscarinic agonist for glaucoma.

Q109. Drug causing mydriasis without cycloplegia?
Phenylephrine
α1 agonist, no effect on accommodation.

Q110. Anti-glaucoma drug causing eyelash growth?
Latanoprost
Not ANS directly, but used ophthalmically.

Q111. Side effect of cholinesterase inhibitors?
Diarrhea, bradycardia, cramps
Due to ↑ ACh.

Q112. β-blockers used post-MI for?
Reduce mortality
Prevent arrhythmias & remodeling.

Q113. Drug-induced bronchospasm seen with?
Non-selective β-blockers
Blocks β2 → bronchoconstriction.

Q114. Parasympathomimetic used in glaucoma?
Carbachol
Decreases IOP by ↑ outflow.

Q115. α1 agonists used for?
Hypotension, nasal congestion
Vasoconstrictors.

Q116. β1 receptor stimulation causes?
Increased HR, force of contraction
Found in heart.

Q117. β2 stimulation in liver causes?
Glycogenolysis
Increases glucose.

Q118. β2 stimulation in uterus?
Relaxation
Used to delay labor.

Q119. α1 stimulation in genitourinary tract?
Contraction of internal sphincter
Promotes urinary retention.

Q120. M3 receptor in bladder causes?
Detrusor contraction
Promotes urination.

Q121. Drug used for overactive bladder?

Oxybutynin

M3 antagonist → reduces detrusor overactivity.

Q122. Adverse effect of atropine in elderly?

Urinary retention and confusion

CNS penetration.

Q123. Parasympatholytic used pre-op to reduce secretions?

Glycopyrrolate

Antimuscarinic, does not cross BBB.

Q124. Which β-blocker has antioxidant property?

Carvedilol

Also has α-blocking activity.

Q125. Drug used for smoking cessation?

Varenicline

Partial agonist at nicotinic receptors.

Q126. Receptor causing vasoconstriction?

α1

Increases peripheral resistance.

Q127. Receptor responsible for GI motility?

M3

Stimulates smooth muscle.

Q128. Which drug mimics ACh at NMJ?

Succinylcholine

Depolarizing neuromuscular blocker.

Q129. Drug causing excessive parasympathetic activation?

Organophosphates

Irreversible AChE inhibitors.

Q130. Long-acting β2 agonist for asthma?

Salmeterol

Used for maintenance therapy.

Q131. Drug of choice for hypertensive crisis in pheochromocytoma?

Phentolamine

Rapid-acting α-blocker.

Q132. β-blocker with shortest half-life?
Esmolol
Ultra-short acting, IV only.

Q133. Indication for β-blockers in hyperthyroidism?
Control symptoms
Reduce tachycardia, tremor, anxiety.

Q134. Muscarinic agonist used in postoperative ileus?
Bethanechol
Stimulates GI motility.

Q135. Action of α2 agonist in brain?
Inhibits sympathetic outflow
Decreases BP.

Q136. β1 selective blockers mnemonic?
A–M: Atenolol, Bisoprolol, Esmolol, etc.
Safer in asthma, COPD.

Q137. Drugs that cause orthostatic hypotension?
α-blockers like prazosin
Due to venodilation.

Q138. Drug with both α- and β-blocking effects?
Labetalol
Used in hypertensive emergencies.

Q139. α1 receptor stimulation in the pupil causes?
Mydriasis
Radial muscle contraction.

Q140. Antimuscarinic side effects mnemonic?
"Dry as bone, hot as hare…"
Classic atropine toxicity.

Q141. Which β-blocker is lipid-soluble?
Propranolol
Crosses BBB → CNS side effects.

Q142. β-blocker used for performance anxiety?
Propranolol
Reduces tremor, palpitations.

Q143. Mechanism of guanethidine?
Inhibits NE release
Obsolete antihypertensive.

Q144. Cholinergic excess symptoms?
SLUDGE
Muscarinic hyperactivity signs.

Q145. Botulinum toxin inhibits?
ACh release
Used in spasticity, dystonia, cosmetics.

Q146. Drug that reverses α1 effects of epinephrine?
Prazosin
Unmasks β2 → vasodilation.

Q147. Sympathomimetic drug not entering CNS?
Phenylephrine
Polar structure.

Q148. Parasympathetic effect on heart?
Slows heart rate
Via M2 receptors.

Q149. Sympathetic effect on GIT?
Decreased motility
Blood redirected to muscles.

Q150. G-protein type for β1 and β2 receptors?
Gs protein
↑ cAMP → various effects.

Q151. G-protein for α1 receptor?
Gq
Activates IP3-DAG pathway → smooth muscle contraction.

Q152. G-protein for α2 receptor?
Gi
Inhibits cAMP → ↓ NE release.

Q153. G-protein for M2 receptor?
Gi
Slows heart rate via vagus.

Q154. G-protein for M3 receptor?
Gq
Increases glandular secretions and smooth muscle tone.

Q155. Adrenergic receptor in adipose tissue?
β3
Stimulates lipolysis.

Q156. Selective α1 antagonist used in BPH?
Tamsulosin
Relieves urinary obstruction.

Q157. β-blocker with α-blocking property?
Carvedilol
Used in CHF and hypertension.

Q158. Muscarinic receptor location in ciliary muscle?
M3
Causes accommodation.

Q159. Which cholinomimetic causes accommodation spasm?
Pilocarpine
M3 stimulation of ciliary muscle.

Q160. Which drug causes dry mouth and constipation?
Atropine
Anticholinergic effect.

Q161. Which drug decreases aqueous humor production?
Timolol
β-blocker for glaucoma.

Q162. Which drug increases outflow of aqueous humor?
Pilocarpine
Constricts ciliary muscle.

Q163. Which receptor causes vasodilation in skeletal muscle?
β2
Seen with low-dose epinephrine.

Q164. Which adrenergic receptor dilates bronchi?
β2
Relaxes bronchial smooth muscle.

Q165. β-blocker useful in hyperthyroid tremor?
Propranolol
Blocks β2 action on muscle spindles.

Q166. Parasympathomimetic for xerostomia?
Cevimeline
Muscarinic agonist used in Sjögren's.

Q167. Drug of choice in atropine-induced delirium?
Physostigmine
Crosses BBB.

Q168. Drug that blocks all muscarinic receptors?
Atropine
Competitive antagonist.

Q169. Which β-blocker causes cold extremities?
Propranolol
↓ peripheral perfusion.

Q170. Which adrenergic drug improves renal perfusion?
Low-dose dopamine
Stimulates D1 receptors.

Q171. α2 agonist that reduces sympathetic outflow?
Methyldopa
Preferred in pregnancy.

Q172. Which anticholinergic is contraindicated in glaucoma?
Atropine
Increases IOP.

Q173. β-blocker with partial agonist action?
Pindolol
Less bradycardia and lipid disturbance.

Q174. Which drug is an indirect sympathomimetic?
Amphetamine
Promotes NE release.

Q175. Which neurotransmitter is in sweat glands?
Acetylcholine
Acts on muscarinic receptors despite being sympathetic.

Q176. M3 receptor in lungs causes?
Bronchoconstriction and ↑ secretions
Opposite of β2 action.

Q177. Adverse effect of ganglion blockers?
Postural hypotension
Due to loss of sympathetic tone.

Q178. Adrenergic drug with dose-dependent receptor effects?
Dopamine
D1 < β1 < α1 (low to high dose sequence).

Q179. Sympathetic preganglionic fibers release?
Acetylcholine
Acts on nicotinic receptors.

Q180. Parasympathetic postganglionic fibers release?
Acetylcholine
Acts on muscarinic receptors.

Q181. Sympathetic postganglionic neurotransmitter (most)?
Norepinephrine
Except in sweat glands (ACh).

Q182. Receptor causing ejaculation?
α1
Smooth muscle contraction.

Q183. Receptor causing penile erection?
M3 (via NO pathway)
Parasympathetic "point" response.

Q184. M2 receptor effect on heart?
Decreases HR and AV conduction
Vagal stimulation.

Q185. β1 effect on heart?
Increases HR, contractility, and AV conduction
Adrenergic effect.

Q186. Which drug causes tachyphylaxis?
Ephedrine
Rapid depletion of NE stores.

Q187. Drug used in atropine poisoning?
Physostigmine
Central and peripheral AChE inhibition.

Q188. Indication for ipratropium?
COPD and asthma
Inhaled muscarinic antagonist.

Q189. Ganglion-blocking drug (obsolete)?
Hexamethonium
Blocks nicotinic receptors at ganglia.

Q190. Cholinergic agonist with no CNS penetration?
Neostigmine
Quaternary structure.

Q191. Contraindication for β-blockers?
Asthma, bradycardia, AV block
Risk of worsening bronchospasm or conduction block.

Q192. Direct muscarinic agonist for urinary retention?
Bethanechol
Selective for bladder and GI tract.

Q193. β-blocker that crosses BBB easily?
Propranolol
Lipid-soluble → CNS effects.

Q194. Drug reducing cardiac oxygen demand?
β-blockers
↓ HR and contractility.

Q195. Antidote for β-blocker overdose?
Glucagon
Increases cAMP via non-β receptors.

Q196. Drug used in postural hypotension?
Midodrine
α1 agonist.

Q197. Muscarinic antagonist causing sedation?
Scopolamine
Crosses BBB.

Q198. Why anticholinergics cause hyperthermia?

↓ Sweat gland activity
Risk of heat stroke in children.

Q199. Succinylcholine metabolism by?

Pseudocholinesterase
Deficiency → prolonged paralysis.

Q200. Drug used to reverse non-depolarizing blockade?

Neostigmine (with atropine)
Inhibits AChE, increases ACh to outcompete blocker.

CVS Pharmacology

Q1. Drug of choice in acute MI?
Aspirin
Antiplatelet action reduces mortality.

Q2. First-line antihypertensive in diabetics?
ACE inhibitors
Renoprotective, reduce proteinuria.

Q3. Drug of choice in hypertensive emergency?
Sodium nitroprusside
Arterial and venous vasodilator.

Q4. Side effect of ACE inhibitors?
Dry cough
Due to ↑ bradykinin.

Q5. Antidote for cyanide toxicity from nitroprusside?
Sodium thiosulfate
Enhances cyanide detoxification.

Q6. Angiotensin receptor blocker (ARB) example?
Losartan
Blocks AT1 receptor.

Q7. Advantage of ARBs over ACE inhibitors?
No cough
Bradykinin is not increased.

Q8. Calcium channel blocker causing constipation?
Verapamil
Non-dihydropyridine with cardiac effects.

Q9. First-line drug in variant (Prinzmetal) angina?
Calcium channel blockers
Relieves coronary vasospasm.

Q10. Nitrate mechanism of action?
↑ NO → ↑ cGMP → vasodilation
Mainly venodilation.

Q11. Nitrate tolerance is prevented by?
Nitrate-free interval
Usually at night.

Q12. Contraindication for nitrates?
Sildenafil use
Risk of severe hypotension.

Q13. β-blockers used in angina act by?
↓ HR and contractility
Reduces myocardial O2 demand.

Q14. Drug contraindicated in variant angina?
β-blockers
May worsen vasospasm.

Q15. DOC in hypertensive crisis in pregnancy?
Labetalol
α and β-blocking activity.

Q16. Direct vasodilator causing hypertrichosis?
Minoxidil
Topical use in alopecia.

Q17. Hydralazine causes?
Arteriolar dilation
Reflex tachycardia and lupus-like syndrome.

Q18. Drug causing drug-induced lupus?
Hydralazine
Especially in slow acetylators.

Q19. Diuretic used in heart failure?
Furosemide
Relieves pulmonary edema.

Q20. Aldosterone antagonist improving survival in CHF?
Spironolactone
↓ Remodeling, ↓ mortality.

Q21. Most potent class of diuretics?
Loop diuretics
Act on thick ascending limb.

Q22. Thiazide diuretics act on?
Distal convoluted tubule
Inhibit Na^+/Cl^- symporter.

Q23. Side effect of thiazides?
Hyperuricemia
Risk of gout.

Q24. β-blocker contraindicated in heart block?
Propranolol
Worsens AV conduction.

Q25. Nifedipine mainly acts on?
Vascular smooth muscle
Dihydropyridine CCB.

Q26. Verapamil effect on AV node?
Slows conduction
Used in supraventricular tachycardia (SVT).

Q27. Antihypertensive causing reflex tachycardia?
Hydralazine
Arteriolar vasodilation.

Q28. K^+ channel opener used in HTN?
Minoxidil
Powerful vasodilator.

Q29. Central α2 agonist antihypertensive?
Clonidine
Reduces sympathetic outflow.

Q30. Clonidine withdrawal causes?
Rebound hypertension
Due to sudden sympathetic surge.

Q31. Loop diuretics inhibit which transporter?
Na^+-K^+-$2Cl^-$ symporter
Located in thick ascending limb.

Q32. Diuretic causing ototoxicity?
Furosemide
Especially with rapid IV push.

Q33. Potassium-sparing diuretic?
Amiloride
Blocks ENaC in collecting duct.

Q34. Diuretic that causes gynecomastia?
Spironolactone
Antiandrogenic side effects.

Q35. Drug class contraindicated in bilateral renal artery stenosis?
ACE inhibitors
Can precipitate renal failure.

Q36. Drug of choice for isolated systolic hypertension in elderly?
Thiazide diuretics
Reduces stroke risk.

Q37. β-blocker used in chronic heart failure?
Metoprolol
Improves long-term outcomes.

Q38. Mechanism of digoxin?
Inhibits Na^+/K^+ ATPase
↑ intracellular Ca^{2+} → ↑ contractility.

Q39. ECG change in digoxin toxicity?
Scooped ST depression
Also causes AV block, ectopics.

Q40. Electrolyte imbalance worsening digoxin toxicity?
Hypokalemia
Enhances digoxin binding to Na^+/K^+ ATPase.

Q41. Antidote for digoxin toxicity?
Digoxin-specific Fab fragments
Bind and neutralize circulating drug.

Q42. Drug causing cyanide toxicity?
Sodium nitroprusside
Monitor in prolonged use.

Q43. Vasodilator that acts via K^+ channel opening?
Minoxidil
Causes hyperpolarization.

Q44. Drug used for hypertrophic cardiomyopathy?
β-blockers
Reduce outflow obstruction and O_2 demand.

Q45. Drug used for rate control in atrial fibrillation?
Diltiazem
Calcium channel blocker (non-DHP).

Q46. Drug of choice in paroxysmal supraventricular tachycardia (PSVT)?
Adenosine
Causes transient AV block.

Q47. Side effect of adenosine?
Flushing, chest pain, bronchospasm
Very short-acting.

Q48. Drug class causing ankle edema?
Dihydropyridine CCBs
Due to arteriolar dilation.

Q49. Short-acting nitrate?
Sublingual nitroglycerin
Used for acute angina relief.

Q50. Long-acting nitrate example?
Isosorbide mononitrate
Used for angina prophylaxis.

Q51. Nitrate-free interval is required to avoid?
Tolerance
Most commonly scheduled overnight.

Q52. Antihypertensive preferred in renal failure with proteinuria?
ACE inhibitors
Reduce intraglomerular pressure.

Q53. Direct renin inhibitor?
Aliskiren
Inhibits conversion of angiotensinogen to Ang I.

Q54. Drug used for angina and also reduces heart rate?
Ivabradine
Selective funny current (If) inhibitor.

Q55. First-line antihypertensive in black patients (without CKD)?
Thiazide diuretics or CCBs
Better BP control.

Q56. Lipid-lowering drug contraindicated in pregnancy?
Statins
Teratogenic.

Q57. Drug of choice for hypertensive crisis + tachycardia?
Labetalol
Combined α and β blockade.

Q58. Side effect of hydralazine?
Drug-induced lupus
More in slow acetylators.

Q59. Which antihypertensive causes hypertrichosis?
Minoxidil
Used topically for alopecia.

Q60. Which class of CCB is preferred for arrhythmias?
Non-dihydropyridines (e.g., verapamil, diltiazem)
Act on cardiac conduction.

Q61. Calcium channel blocker safest in heart failure?
Amlodipine
Least negative inotropic effect among CCBs.

Q62. Effect of verapamil on AV node?
Decreases conduction
Used for supraventricular arrhythmias.

Q63. Effect of nifedipine on heart rate?
Reflex tachycardia
Due to vasodilation and BP drop.

Q64. CCB that may worsen heart failure?
Verapamil
Due to negative inotropic effect.

Q65. Lipid-lowering drug causing flushing?
Niacin
Due to prostaglandin-mediated vasodilation.

Q66. Drug used to prevent niacin flushing?
Aspirin (low dose)
Inhibits prostaglandins.

Q67. Statins inhibit which enzyme?
HMG-CoA reductase
Key enzyme in cholesterol synthesis.

Q68. Main side effect of statins?
Myopathy
Also monitor liver enzymes.

Q69. Drug class used for isolated hypertriglyceridemia?
Fibrates
Activate PPAR-α → ↑ LPL activity.

Q70. Drug increasing HDL the most?
Niacin
Also lowers LDL and TG.

Q71. Drug binding bile acids in intestine?
Cholestyramine
Causes GI side effects and drug malabsorption.

Q72. Statins are most effective for?
Lowering LDL
First-line for atherosclerosis.

Q73. Fibrate side effect with statin use?
Myopathy risk ↑
Use with caution.

Q74. PCSK9 inhibitors action?
Prevent LDL receptor degradation
↑ LDL clearance (e.g., evolocumab).

Q75. Omega-3 fatty acids effect on lipids?
↓ Triglycerides
Mild effect on HDL/LDL.

Q76. Anti-anginal drug that does not affect HR or BP?
Ranolazine
Inhibits late Na^+ current.

Q77. Which nitrate has high first-pass metabolism?
Isosorbide dinitrate (oral)
Not effective sublingually.

Q78. Drug contraindicated with PDE-5 inhibitors?
Nitrates
Severe hypotension risk.

Q79. Common adverse effect of nitrates?
Headache
Due to meningeal vasodilation.

Q80. Nitrate effect on preload?
Decreases
Via venodilation.

Q81. Drugs causing reflex tachycardia?
Nifedipine, hydralazine
Due to drop in BP.

Q82. Ivabradine mechanism of action?
Inhibits funny current (If) in SA node
Slows HR without affecting BP.

Q83. First-line antihypertensive in CKD with proteinuria?
ACE inhibitors
Protects against nephropathy.

Q84. Drug that worsens hyperkalemia in CKD?
Spironolactone
Avoid or monitor K^+ levels.

Q85. Loop diuretic effect on calcium?
Hypocalcemia
Blocks paracellular reabsorption.

Q86. Thiazide diuretic effect on calcium?
Hypercalcemia
Enhances distal tubular Ca^{2+} reabsorption.

Q87. Drug of choice for atrial fibrillation with rapid rate?
Diltiazem or β-blockers
Slow AV node conduction.

Q88. Anticoagulant used in atrial fibrillation?
Apixaban (DOAC) or warfarin
Prevents thromboembolism.

Q89. Side effect of spironolactone in males?
Gynecomastia
Antiandrogenic property.

Q90. Drug causing "lupus-like" syndrome?
Hydralazine
Especially in slow acetylators.

Q91. Diuretic useful in nephrolithiasis due to hypercalciuria?
Thiazide
Decreases calcium excretion in urine.

Q92. Loop diuretics used in?
Pulmonary edema
Rapid action and strong diuresis.

Q93. Diuretic safe in lithium-induced diabetes insipidus?
Amiloride
Blocks ENaC, reduces lithium uptake.

Q94. β-blocker with highest cardioselectivity?
Bisoprolol
β1-selective, minimal β2 effect.

Q95. β-blocker with nitric oxide-mediated vasodilation?
Nebivolol
Also improves endothelial function.

Q96. Drug of choice in acute decompensated heart failure?
Dobutamine
β1 agonist → inotropic support.

Q97. Phosphodiesterase-3 inhibitor in HF?
Milrinone
Increases cAMP → inotropic + vasodilation.

Q98. ACE inhibitors cause hyperkalemia due to?
↓ Aldosterone
Leads to K^+ retention.

Q99. Statins are contraindicated with which antibiotic?
Erythromycin
Increases statin levels → myopathy.

Q100. Ivabradine does not affect?
Blood pressure
Pure HR lowering agent.

Q101. Antianginal drug safe in hypotension?
Ivabradine
Does not cause vasodilation.

Q102. Drug that prolongs QT but is used in angina?
Ranolazine
Monitor ECG during use.

Q103. Drug used for cyanide poisoning?
Hydroxocobalamin
Preferred over older nitrites.

Q104. ACE inhibitor fetotoxicity occurs in?
2nd and 3rd trimesters
Can cause oligohydramnios, fetal renal failure.

Q105. ACE inhibitors cause which renal effect?
Efferent arteriole vasodilation
↓ GFR especially in bilateral renal artery stenosis.

Q106. Thiazide effect on uric acid?
Increases
Risk of gout.

Q107. β-blocker used in dissecting aneurysm?
Esmolol
Rapid action and short half-life.

Q108. Adverse effect of dobutamine?
Arrhythmia
Due to β1 stimulation.

Q109. Milrinone side effect?
Ventricular arrhythmias
cAMP-mediated effect.

Q110. Osmotic diuretic example?
Mannitol
Used in cerebral edema.

Q111. Contraindication to mannitol?
CHF
Can cause pulmonary edema.

Q112. Drug class causing hyperkalemia?
K^+-sparing diuretics
Especially with ACE inhibitors.

Q113. Potassium-wasting diuretics?
Loop and thiazide diuretics
Can lead to hypokalemia.

Q114. Adverse effect of statins with gemfibrozil?
Rhabdomyolysis
Avoid this combination.

Q115. Statins most commonly elevate which enzyme?
ALT
Indicates hepatotoxicity.

Q116. Ezetimibe mechanism of action?
Inhibits cholesterol absorption
At intestinal brush border.

Q117. Bile acid resin that raises TGs?
Cholestyramine
Contraindicated in hypertriglyceridemia.

Q118. Drug that inhibits hepatic VLDL secretion?
Niacin
Also raises HDL.

Q119. Statin metabolized via CYP3A4?
Atorvastatin
Drug interaction risk ↑.

Q120. LDL-lowering therapy in familial hypercholesterolemia?
PCSK9 inhibitors
Monoclonal antibodies.

Q121. Antihypertensive causing hyperprolactinemia?
Verapamil
Inhibits dopamine release → ↑ prolactin.

Q122. Shortest-acting calcium channel blocker?
Clevidipine
Used IV in hypertensive emergencies.

Q123. Dihydropyridine CCB with reflex tachycardia?
Nifedipine
Potent vasodilator, minimal cardiac effect.

Q124. Drug of choice in hypertension + BPH?
Prazosin
α1-blocker → lowers BP and improves urine flow.

Q125. Major side effect of α1 blockers?
Postural hypotension
Especially with first dose.

Q126. Diuretic class that increases serum calcium?
Thiazides
Enhances distal Ca^{2+} reabsorption.

Q127. Drug that reduces both preload and afterload?
Nitroprusside
Balanced arterial and venous dilator.

Q128. Fenoldopam mechanism?
D1 agonist
Vasodilation + natriuresis.

Q129. Drug used to control bleeding from esophageal varices?
Propranolol
Non-selective β-blocker → ↓ portal pressure.

Q130. Oral nitrate used for angina prophylaxis?
Isosorbide mononitrate
Long-acting agent.

Q131. Drug for prevention of sudden cardiac death post-MI?
β-blockers
↓ Arrhythmic risk and mortality.

Q132. Antiarrhythmic drug that also lowers BP and HR?
Verapamil
CCB with cardiac selectivity.

Q133. Renin inhibitor used in hypertension?
Aliskiren
Blocks RAAS at its source.

Q134. Antihypertensive to avoid in pregnancy?
ACE inhibitors
Risk of fetal renal damage.

Q135. Antihypertensive safe in pregnancy?
Methyldopa
Central $\alpha 2$ agonist.

Q136. CCB preferred in pregnancy?
Nifedipine
Used for BP and tocolysis.

Q137. Drug that increases natriuretic peptides?
Sacubitril
Combined with valsartan in HF.

Q138. Role of valsartan in ARNI combo?
Blocks AT1 receptors
Prevents angiotensin II effects.

Q139. Nesiritide is analog of?
BNP
Causes vasodilation and natriuresis.

Q140. Side effect of nesiritide?
Hypotension
Used in acute decompensated HF.

Q141. Dopamine receptor causing renal vasodilation?
D1
Low dose improves perfusion.

Q142. Milrinone effect on vasculature?
Vasodilation
PDE-3 inhibition increases cAMP.

Q143. Drug used for cyanide toxicity from nitroprusside?
Sodium thiosulfate
Converts cyanide to thiocyanate.

Q144. Drug with "antihypertensive + hair growth" effect?
Minoxidil
K^+ channel opener.

Q145. Drug contraindicated with statins?
Gemfibrozil
↑ Risk of myopathy.

Q146. Most potent LDL-lowering agent?
PCSK9 inhibitors
Monoclonal antibody.

Q147. LDL receptor synthesis ↑ by?
Statins
Compensatory upregulation.

Q148. HDL increase best with?
Niacin
Also ↓ LDL and TG.

Q149. TG-lowering drug activating LPL?
Fibrates
Via PPAR-α activation.

Q150. Statin benefit in coronary artery disease?
Plaque stabilization
↓ Inflammation and thrombosis risk.

Q151. Most common side effect of loop diuretics?
Hypokalemia
Due to increased K^+ excretion.

Q152. Antihypertensive safe in asthma?
Amlodipine
CCBs have no bronchoconstrictive effect.

Q153. CCB contraindicated in heart failure?
Verapamil
Negative inotrope.

Q154. Amiodarone acts on which class?
Class III (K^+ channel blocker)
Also has Class I, II, IV effects.

Q155. Major toxicity of amiodarone?
Pulmonary fibrosis
Also causes thyroid dysfunction, liver toxicity.

Q156. Drug that prolongs QT but has low torsades risk?
Amiodarone
Unique property among Class III agents.

Q157. Sotalol class of antiarrhythmic?
Class III
Also has β-blocker effect.

Q158. Drug used in torsades de pointes?
Magnesium sulfate
Stabilizes cardiac membrane.

Q159. Drug class that shortens action potential duration?
Class IB (e.g., lidocaine)
Especially in ischemic tissue.

Q160. Antiarrhythmic causing lupus-like syndrome?
Procainamide
Class IA drug.

Q161. Flecainide class?
Class IC
Potent Na^+ channel blocker.

Q162. Adenosine acts on?
A1 receptors in AV node
Causes transient heart block.

Q163. Side effect of adenosine?
Flushing, bronchospasm, chest discomfort
Very short half-life.

Q164. β-blocker antiarrhythmic class?
Class II
Decrease slope of phase 4 in pacemaker cells.

Q165. Drug causing thyrotoxicosis and hypothyroidism?
Amiodarone
Contains iodine.

Q166. Class of verapamil as antiarrhythmic?
Class IV
CCB acting on AV node.

Q167. Preferred drug for rate control in atrial flutter?
Diltiazem
Non-DHP CCB.

Q168. Digoxin toxicity ECG feature?
PVCs, AV block, scooped ST
High-dose effect.

Q169. Effect of digoxin on AV conduction?
Slows
Useful in AF with HF.

Q170. Effect of hyperkalemia on digoxin action?
Reduces toxicity
Competes with digoxin binding.

Q171. Ivabradine acts on?
Funny current (If)
Slows SA node without BP drop.

Q172. Antiarrhythmic that prolongs PR interval?
β-blockers and non-DHP CCBs
Slow AV node conduction.

Q173. Class I antiarrhythmics act on which phase?
Phase 0
Na^+ channel blockade.

Q174. Class III antiarrhythmics act on which phase?
Phase 3
K^+ channel blockade → prolonged repolarization.

Q175. Main side effect of quinidine?
Cinchonism
Tinnitus, headache, blurred vision.

Q176. Drug contraindicated in WPW syndrome with AF?
Verapamil
Can increase conduction via accessory pathway.

Q177. Amiodarone half-life?
Very long (~50 days)
Requires loading dose.

Q178. Drug causing blue-grey skin pigmentation?
Amiodarone
Also phototoxicity.

Q179. Antiarrhythmic contraindicated in structural heart disease?
Flecainide
Risk of proarrhythmia.

Q180. Class IB drug used in post-MI arrhythmia?
Lidocaine
Prefers ischemic myocardium.

Q181. Lidocaine route of administration?
IV
Poor oral bioavailability.

Q182. Class IC drugs affect which part of the ECG?
QRS widening
Due to potent Na^+ channel block.

Q183. β-blocker used IV for rapid rate control?
Esmolol
Ultra-short acting.

Q184. Sotalol side effect?
Torsades de pointes
Prolongs QT interval.

Q185. Class IA drugs effect on action potential duration?
Prolonged
Also increase QT interval.

Q186. Lidocaine selectively targets?
Ischemic ventricular tissue
Makes it useful in post-MI arrhythmias.

Q187. Drug causing bronchospasm in COPD?
Non-selective β-blockers
e.g., propranolol.

Q188. Diuretic used in resistant hypertension?
Chlorthalidone
Long-acting thiazide-like agent.

Q189. Drug safe in pregnancy-induced hypertension?
Methyldopa
Centrally acting α2 agonist.

Q190. Oral drug for chronic angina not affecting BP or HR?
Ranolazine
Late Na^+ current inhibitor.

Q191. Amiodarone thyroid side effect mechanism?
Iodine content
Can cause hypo- or hyperthyroidism.

Q192. Which antiarrhythmic increases digoxin level?
Quinidine
Displaces digoxin from tissue binding.

Q193. Nitrate tolerance due to?
Depletion of sulfhydryl groups
Need nitrate-free interval.

Q194. Class III drug that causes QT prolongation with low torsades risk?
Amiodarone
Safer despite prolonged repolarization.

Q195. Drug that enhances baroreceptor sensitivity?
Clonidine
Central sympatholytic.

Q196. β-blocker that also causes vasodilation via NO?
Nebivolol
Dual mechanism.

Q197. Heart failure drug combination reducing mortality?
Sacubitril + Valsartan (ARNI)
Enhances natriuretic peptides + blocks RAAS.

Q198. Digoxin effect on intracellular calcium?

Increases

Via Na^+/K^+ ATPase inhibition.

Q199. Drug used in digitalis-induced arrhythmias?

Lidocaine

Suppresses ventricular ectopics.

Q200. Drug used for hypertensive urgency (oral)?

Captopril

Quick onset, short-acting ACE inhibitor.

CNS Pharmacology

Q1. Main excitatory neurotransmitter in CNS?
Glutamate
Acts via NMDA and AMPA receptors.

Q2. Main inhibitory neurotransmitter in CNS?
GABA
Acts on GABA-A (Cl^- channel) and GABA-B (GPCR).

Q3. Mechanism of benzodiazepines?
Enhance GABA-A receptor activity
Increase frequency of Cl^- channel opening.

Q4. Mechanism of barbiturates?
Enhance GABA-A receptor activity
Increase duration of Cl^- channel opening.

Q5. Benzodiazepine with shortest half-life?
Midazolam
Used for induction and conscious sedation.

Q6. Long-acting benzodiazepine?
Diazepam
Used for seizures, anxiety, alcohol withdrawal.

Q7. Antidote for benzodiazepine overdose?
Flumazenil
Competitive GABA-A antagonist.

Q8. Barbiturate with high anticonvulsant effect?
Phenobarbital
Also induces CYP450 enzymes.

Q9. Anesthetic with rapid induction and recovery?
Propofol
Enhances GABA-A activity.

Q10. Propofol infusion syndrome includes?
Metabolic acidosis, rhabdomyolysis
Rare but fatal.

Q11. IV anesthetic causing dissociative anesthesia?
Ketamine
NMDA antagonist, increases BP and HR.

Q12. Hallucinations and emergence delirium caused by?
Ketamine
More in adults.

Q13. Inhalational anesthetic with least blood solubility?
Nitrous oxide
Fast onset and recovery.

Q14. Inhalational anesthetic causing hepatotoxicity?
Halothane
Immune-mediated.

Q15. Malignant hyperthermia triggered by?
Succinylcholine + volatile anesthetics
Genetic predisposition.

Q16. Drug of choice for malignant hyperthermia?
Dantrolene
Inhibits ryanodine receptor → ↓ Ca^{2+}.

Q17. DOC for absence seizures?
Ethosuximide
Blocks T-type Ca^{2+} channels in thalamus.

Q18. Drug for generalized tonic-clonic and partial seizures?
Valproic acid
Also used for bipolar and migraine prophylaxis.

Q19. Valproate side effects?
Hepatotoxicity, neural tube defects
Avoid in pregnancy.

Q20. Na^+ channel blocker used for focal seizures?
Carbamazepine
Also DOC for trigeminal neuralgia.

Q21. Carbamazepine side effects?
SIADH, aplastic anemia, rash
CYP450 inducer.

Q22. Antiepileptic causing gingival hyperplasia?
Phenytoin
Also causes hirsutism, ataxia.

Q23. Phenytoin mechanism?
Na^+ channel inactivation
Prevents repetitive firing.

Q24. Antiepileptic with minimal sedation?
Lamotrigine
Na^+ channel blocker, broad-spectrum.

Q25. Lamotrigine side effect?
Stevens–Johnson syndrome
Especially with rapid dose escalation.

Q26. Broad-spectrum antiepileptic safe in liver disease?
Levetiracetam
Binds SV2A → modulates neurotransmitter release.

Q27. Gabapentin mechanism?
Inhibits voltage-gated Ca^{2+} channels
Used in neuropathic pain.

Q28. Topiramate uses?
Seizures, migraine, weight loss
Carbonic anhydrase inhibition.

Q29. Benzodiazepine used in status epilepticus?
Lorazepam
Preferred over diazepam due to longer CNS duration.

Q30. Drug used in febrile seizures?
Diazepam (rectal)
Rapid CNS penetration.

Q31. Parkinson's disease is due to deficiency of?
Dopamine
Especially in substantia nigra pars compacta.

Q32. Levodopa is converted to dopamine by?
DOPA decarboxylase
Occurs peripherally and centrally.

Q33. Why carbidopa is given with levodopa?
Inhibits peripheral DOPA decarboxylase
↑ CNS availability of levodopa.

Q34. Side effect of levodopa?
Dyskinesia, hallucinations
More common with long-term use.

Q35. COMT inhibitor used in Parkinson's?
Entacapone
Prolongs levodopa action.

Q36. MAO-B inhibitor in Parkinson's?
Selegiline
↓ Dopamine breakdown.

Q37. Dopamine agonist causing impulse control disorder?
Pramipexole
Non-ergot, also used in restless leg syndrome.

Q38. Antiviral used in Parkinson's?
Amantadine
↑ dopamine release, ↓ reuptake.

Q39. Drug causing livedo reticularis?
Amantadine
Reticulated skin discoloration.

Q40. Anticholinergic used for tremor in Parkinson's?
Benztropine
Avoid in elderly due to cognitive side effects.

Q41. Alzheimer's disease associated neurotransmitter?
↓ Acetylcholine
Especially in nucleus basalis of Meynert.

Q42. Acetylcholinesterase inhibitor for Alzheimer's?
Donepezil
Improves cognition modestly.

Q43. NMDA receptor antagonist in Alzheimer's?
Memantine
Used in moderate to severe disease.

Q44. Drug class used in acute migraine?
Triptans
5-HT1B/1D agonists → cranial vasoconstriction.

Q45. Triptan side effect?
Chest tightness
Contraindicated in CAD.

Q46. Prophylaxis of migraine includes?
Propranolol, topiramate, valproate
Taken daily to prevent attacks.

Q47. DOC for acute cluster headache?
Oxygen + sumatriptan
Inhaled O_2 aborts attack rapidly.

Q48. Drug used in serotonin syndrome?
Cyproheptadine
5-HT2A antagonist.

Q49. First-line drug for generalized anxiety disorder?
SSRIs (e.g., sertraline)
Safer long-term profile.

Q50. Benzodiazepine preferred in liver disease?
Lorazepam
Not metabolized by CYP450.

Q51. SSRI causing sexual dysfunction?
Fluoxetine
Also causes insomnia.

Q52. SNRI example?
Venlafaxine
Used in depression and neuropathic pain.

Q53. Antidepressant with least sexual side effects?
Bupropion
Also used for smoking cessation.

Q54. Bupropion contraindicated in?
Seizure disorder, eating disorders
Lowers seizure threshold.

Q55. Atypical antidepressant with weight gain + sedation?
Mirtazapine
H1 and α2 antagonist.

Q56. TCA overdose complication?
Cardiotoxicity (QRS prolongation)
Due to Na^+ channel blockade.

Q57. Antidote for TCA overdose?
Sodium bicarbonate
Alkalinizes plasma, stabilizes myocardium.

Q58. MAOI + tyramine causes?
Hypertensive crisis
Tyramine displaces NE.

Q59. Drug interaction of SSRIs with MAOIs?
Serotonin syndrome
Never combine without washout.

Q60. Longest-acting SSRI?
Fluoxetine
Washout needed before MAOI initiation.

Q61. Lithium is used in?
Bipolar disorder
Mood stabilizer, prevents mania & depression.

Q62. Major toxicity of lithium?
Nephrogenic diabetes insipidus
Due to ADH resistance.

Q63. Lithium excretion is affected by?
Sodium levels
Hyponatremia increases lithium reabsorption.

Q64. Drug causing Ebstein anomaly in fetus?
Lithium
Tricuspid valve abnormality.

Q65. Drug of choice for lithium toxicity?
Hemodialysis
Especially in severe neurotoxicity or renal failure.

Q66. Mood stabilizer safe in pregnancy?
Lamotrigine
Lowest teratogenic risk.

Q67. Antipsychotic class causing extrapyramidal symptoms (EPS)?
Typical antipsychotics
Especially high-potency like haloperidol.

Q68. Antipsychotic with least EPS?
Clozapine
Atypical; causes agranulocytosis.

Q69. Antipsychotic causing highest weight gain?
Olanzapine
Also causes sedation and metabolic syndrome.

Q70. Atypical antipsychotic that increases prolactin?
Risperidone
Blocks D2 strongly.

Q71. Dopamine pathway causing EPS when blocked?
Nigrostriatal pathway
Involved in movement control.

Q72. Dopamine pathway responsible for antipsychotic efficacy?
Mesolimbic pathway
Positive symptoms reduced.

Q73. Dopamine pathway linked to negative symptoms?
Mesocortical pathway
Blockade may worsen these symptoms.

Q74. Hyperprolactinemia due to blockade of?
Tuberoinfundibular pathway
↓ dopamine → ↑ prolactin.

Q75. Drug of choice for acute dystonia?
Benztropine
Anticholinergic; reverses EPS.

Q76. Drug used for neuroleptic malignant syndrome (NMS)?
Dantrolene or bromocriptine
NMS = rigidity, fever, ↑ CK.

Q77. Life-threatening antipsychotic complication?
Neuroleptic malignant syndrome
Differentiated from serotonin syndrome by "lead-pipe" rigidity.

Q78. Clozapine requires monitoring for?
Agranulocytosis
Weekly CBC in early treatment.

Q79. SGA with lowest metabolic side effects?
Aripiprazole
Partial D2 agonist.

Q80. Antipsychotic safe in Parkinson's disease psychosis?
Quetiapine
Least motor side effects.

Q81. SGA with highest risk of QT prolongation?
Ziprasidone
Caution in cardiac patients.

Q82. Atypical antipsychotic that is partial D2 agonist?
Aripiprazole
Also used for depression augmentation.

Q83. High-potency typical antipsychotics?
Haloperidol, fluphenazine
↑ EPS risk.

Q84. Low-potency typical antipsychotic with anticholinergic effects?
Chlorpromazine
Causes sedation and orthostatic hypotension.

Q85. Antipsychotic used in Tourette syndrome?
Haloperidol
Controls tics.

Q86. Antipsychotic used for refractory schizophrenia?
Clozapine
Most effective but risky.

Q87. Drugs causing tardive dyskinesia?
Long-term dopamine blockers
Often irreversible.

Q88. Antipsychotic least likely to cause tardive dyskinesia?
Clozapine
Minimal D2 blockade in striatum.

Q89. Drug used in acute mania?
Valproic acid
Rapid mood stabilization.

Q90. Drug with both antipsychotic and mood stabilizer roles?
Quetiapine
Approved for bipolar depression.

Q91. CNS stimulant used in ADHD?
Methylphenidate
Blocks dopamine and NE reuptake.

Q92. Non-stimulant for ADHD?
Atomoxetine
Selective NE reuptake inhibitor.

Q93. Narcolepsy treatment drug?
Modafinil
Promotes wakefulness; mechanism not fully known.

Q94. Acamprosate use?
Alcohol abstinence maintenance
NMDA antagonist.

Q95. Disulfiram mechanism?
Inhibits aldehyde dehydrogenase
Causes acetaldehyde accumulation → aversion.

Q96. Naltrexone use in addiction?
Opioid and alcohol dependence
Blocks reward pathway.

Q97. Opioid receptor with euphoria?
Mu (μ) receptor
Most abused opioids act here.

Q98. Opioid used for diarrhea?
Loperamide
Peripheral action only, no CNS effect.

Q99. Opioid antagonist for overdose?
Naloxone
Fast-acting, IV or intranasal.

Q100. Long-acting opioid antagonist?
Naltrexone
Used in maintenance therapy.

Q101. Partial μ-agonist used in de-addiction?
Buprenorphine
Ceiling effect limits respiratory depression.

Q102. Opioid causing serotonin syndrome?
Meperidine
Avoid with MAO inhibitors.

Q103. Opioid safe in biliary colic?
Meperidine
Less sphincter of Oddi spasm.

Q104. Opioid with cough suppressant effect?
Codeine
Mild μ-agonist.

Q105. Tramadol caution due to?
Seizure risk
Also inhibits 5-HT and NE reuptake.

Q106. Tolerance develops least to which opioid effect?
Constipation & miosis
Persist with chronic use.

Q107. Most dangerous side effect of opioids?
Respiratory depression
Dose-limiting and fatal in overdose.

Q108. Local anesthetic mechanism?
Blocks voltage-gated Na^+ channels
Prevents nerve depolarization.

Q109. Which fibers are blocked first by LA?
Small, unmyelinated (pain)
Size and myelination determine susceptibility.

Q110. LA used topically for mucosal anesthesia?
Benzocaine
Often in lozenges and sprays.

Q111. LA with high cardiotoxicity?
Bupivacaine
Avoid large IV doses.

Q112. LA safest in pregnancy (epidural)?
Ropivacaine
Less motor block and cardiotoxicity.

Q113. Epinephrine is added to LA for?
Prolonging action, reducing toxicity
Vasoconstriction ↓ systemic absorption.

Q114. General anesthetic causing adrenal suppression?
Etomidate
Minimal CV effects but inhibits cortisol synthesis.

Q115. Drug of choice for ECT anesthesia?
Methohexital
Short-acting barbiturate.

Q116. Muscle relaxant with shortest onset?
Succinylcholine
Rapid depolarization block.

Q117. Side effect of succinylcholine?
Hyperkalemia
Risk in burns, trauma, neuromuscular diseases.

Q118. Reversal of non-depolarizing neuromuscular blockers?
Neostigmine
Usually combined with atropine or glycopyrrolate.

Q119. Reversal agent for rocuronium?
Sugammadex
Encapsulates drug; no cholinergic side effects.

Q120. Anticonvulsant safe in pregnancy?
Levetiracetam
Low teratogenic risk, minimal interactions.

Q121. Drug class used in generalized tonic-clonic seizures (GTC)?
Valproate, phenytoin, levetiracetam
All reduce neuronal excitability via Na^+ or Ca^{2+} channels.

Q122. Status epilepticus second-line drug after benzodiazepines?
Phenytoin (or fosphenytoin)
IV loading dose preferred.

Q123. Broad-spectrum antiepileptic safe in elderly?
Levetiracetam
Minimal interactions, no hepatic metabolism.

Q124. Antiepileptic useful in bipolar disorder also?
Valproate
Especially for acute mania.

Q125. Gabapentin is structurally related to?
GABA
But does not act on GABA receptors directly.

Q126. Antiepileptic with risk of hyponatremia?
Carbamazepine
Causes SIADH.

Q127. DOC for trigeminal neuralgia?
Carbamazepine
High efficacy in neuropathic facial pain.

Q128. Lamotrigine acts on?
Voltage-gated Na^+ channels
Delays neuronal repolarization.

Q129. First-line antiepileptic in pregnancy (if needed)?
Levetiracetam or lamotrigine
Lower teratogenic risk.

Q130. Valproate teratogenic effect?
Neural tube defects
Avoid during 1st trimester.

Q131. AED with risk of rash if dose increased too fast?
Lamotrigine
Risk of Stevens-Johnson syndrome.

Q132. Topiramate's dual action?
Blocks Na^+ channels & ↑ GABA
Also inhibits carbonic anhydrase.

Q133. AED causing kidney stones and cognitive slowing?
Topiramate
Common in long-term therapy.

Q134. AED with hepatotoxicity in children <2 years?
Valproate
Requires close monitoring of LFTs.

Q135. AED safe in hepatic failure?
Levetiracetam
Renally excreted.

Q136. GABA-A agonist used for sedation, seizures, anxiety?
Diazepam
Long-acting benzodiazepine.

Q137. Benzodiazepine used in panic disorder?
Alprazolam
Short-acting, high abuse potential.

Q138. Barbiturate used in neonatal seizures?
Phenobarbital
Preferred due to safety profile in neonates.

Q139. DOC for alcohol withdrawal seizures?
Lorazepam
Intermediate-acting BZD, no liver dependence.

Q140. Drug used to prevent relapse in opioid dependence?
Naltrexone
Blocks reward from opioid use.

Q141. Antidepressant safe in sexual dysfunction-prone patients?
Bupropion
No serotonergic activity.

Q142. Antidepressant used for smoking cessation?
Bupropion
Dopamine/NE reuptake inhibitor.

Q143. Serotonin syndrome triad?
Autonomic instability, neuromuscular symptoms, mental status changes
Often drug interaction-related.

Q144. MAO-B inhibitor used in Parkinson's?
Selegiline
Selectively increases dopamine in CNS.

Q145. Antidepressant preferred in underweight and elderly?
Mirtazapine
Appetite stimulant + sedative.

Q146. TCA with least anticholinergic effects?
Nortriptyline
Safer in elderly.

Q147. CNS drug causing hypertensive crisis with cheese/wine?
MAO inhibitors (e.g., tranylcypromine)
Due to tyramine accumulation.

Q148. Longest-acting benzodiazepine?
Diazepam
Half-life up to 100 hours.

Q149. Antipsychotic with both D2 and 5-HT2A antagonism?
Risperidone
Helps both positive and negative symptoms.

Q150. Drug used for sleep-onset insomnia only?
Zaleplon
Short-acting non-BZD hypnotic.

Q151. Non-benzodiazepine hypnotic with minimal hangover effect?
Zolpidem
Acts on BZD-1 receptor → short duration.

Q152. Melatonin receptor agonist for insomnia?
Ramelteon
Targets MT1 and MT2 receptors.

Q153. Drug approved for narcolepsy with cataplexy?
Sodium oxybate (GHB)
Reduces daytime sleep attacks.

Q154. Orexin antagonist used in insomnia?
Suvorexant
Promotes sleep initiation and maintenance.

Q155. Most commonly used inhaled anesthetic today?
Sevoflurane
Low blood solubility, rapid onset and recovery.

Q156. Inhalational anesthetic with highest blood-gas partition coefficient?
Halothane
Slowest onset and recovery.

Q157. Inhaled anesthetic with least myocardial depression?
Desflurane
Stable CV profile.

Q158. Inhalational anesthetic safe in asthma?
Sevoflurane
Non-irritant to airways.

Q159. Inhaled anesthetic with strong pungency and airway irritation?
Desflurane
Not preferred for induction.

Q160. IV anesthetic causing dissociative anesthesia?
Ketamine
NMDA antagonist; maintains airway reflexes.

Q161. Anesthetic with strong analgesic property?
Ketamine
Unlike most other anesthetics.

Q162. Shortest-acting barbiturate for anesthesia induction?
Thiopental
Redistributes quickly to fat and muscle.

Q163. IV anesthetic with least hangover effect?
Propofol
Fast recovery due to rapid hepatic metabolism.

Q164. Drug causing euphoria and hallucinations in anesthesia?
Ketamine
Emergence reactions seen.

Q165. Succinylcholine is contraindicated in?
Burn patients, neuromuscular diseases
Risk of hyperkalemia.

Q166. Non-depolarizing muscle relaxant example?
Vecuronium
Competitive Nm blocker.

Q167. LA used in spinal anesthesia with long duration?
Bupivacaine
Risk of cardiotoxicity if given IV.

Q168. Local anesthetic metabolized by plasma cholinesterase?
Procaine
Ester-type LA.

Q169. LA with hepatic metabolism?
Lidocaine
Amide-type LA.

Q170. Spinal anesthesia blocks which fibers first?
Sympathetic > Pain > Touch > Motor
Due to fiber diameter and myelination.

Q171. Antidepressant also used in chronic pain?
Amitriptyline
TCA with dual analgesic benefit.

Q172. Neuropathic pain drug also used in fibromyalgia?
Pregabalin
Binds $\alpha 2\delta$ subunit of Ca^{2+} channels.

Q173. Drug used in postherpetic neuralgia?
Gabapentin
Effective for neuropathic pain.

Q174. Mechanism of action of baclofen?
GABA-B receptor agonist
Muscle relaxant in spasticity.

Q175. Drug for muscle spasm post-spinal cord injury?
Tizanidine
$\alpha 2$ agonist acting centrally.

Q176. CNS stimulant causing insomnia and anxiety?
Amphetamines
↑ NE and dopamine release.

Q177. Hallucinogen with 5-HT2A agonism?
LSD
Causes altered perception and mood.

Q178. Drug class of phencyclidine (PCP)?
NMDA receptor antagonist
Produces violent behavior and nystagmus.

Q179. Cannabis acts on which receptor?
CB1 receptor
CNS effects (mood, appetite, perception).

Q180. Substance causing conjunctival injection and munchies?
Marijuana
Classic cannabinoid effects.

Q181. DOC for benzodiazepine withdrawal seizures?
Diazepam
Long-acting BZD used to taper dependence.

Q182. Antipsychotic safest for elderly with dementia-related psychosis?
Quetiapine
Lower risk of EPS and sedation.

Q183. Antidepressant causing least sexual dysfunction?
Bupropion
No serotonergic activity.

Q184. MOA of varenicline (smoking cessation drug)?
Partial agonist at nicotinic receptors
Reduces cravings and reward.

Q185. Substance causing pinpoint pupils, respiratory depression?
Opioids (e.g., heroin)
Classic toxidrome of overdose.

Q186. Withdrawal from which drug causes seizures, tremors, hallucinations?
Alcohol
Especially in chronic heavy use.

Q187. Antidepressant with risk of priapism?
Trazodone
Also causes sedation and orthostatic hypotension.

Q188. Anxiolytic with no sedative or dependence risk?
Buspirone
5-HT1A partial agonist, slow onset.

Q189. MOA of modafinil?
Unclear, likely ↑ dopamine
Used for narcolepsy, shift work disorder.

Q190. Street drug with bruxism, hyperthermia, hyponatremia?
MDMA (Ecstasy)
Causes serotonin syndrome-like toxicity.

Q191. Long-term phenytoin use affects bone by?
Causing osteomalacia
Due to ↓ vitamin D metabolism.

Q192. DOC for generalized anxiety disorder (GAD)?
SSRIs or SNRIs
Safer than benzodiazepines long-term.

Q193. Antidepressant with greatest QT prolongation?
Citalopram
Monitor ECG at high doses.

Q194. Antipsychotic causing corneal deposits?
Chlorpromazine
Seen with long-term use.

Q195. Antipsychotic causing retinal pigmentation?
Thioridazine
Leads to vision changes.

Q196. Hallucinogen associated with flashbacks?
LSD
Hallucinogen persisting perception disorder (HPPD).

Q197. Parkinsonian side effect of antipsychotics is due to?
D2 blockade in nigrostriatal tract
EPS develops over weeks.

Q198. Dopaminergic pathway causing positive schizophrenia symptoms?
Mesolimbic
D2 blockade improves hallucinations/delusions.

Q199. AED causing SJS in HLA-B 1502 positive individuals?
Carbamazepine
Screen in Asian populations.

Q200. Antiepileptic that inhibits synaptic vesicle protein SV2A?
Levetiracetam
Broad-spectrum, well tolerated.

Endocrine Pharmacology

Q1. Drug of choice in adrenal insufficiency?
Hydrocortisone
Provides both glucocorticoid and mineralocorticoid activity.

Q2. Long-acting glucocorticoid with no mineralocorticoid effect?
Dexamethasone
Preferred in cerebral edema.

Q3. Most potent mineralocorticoid?
Fludrocortisone
Used in Addison's disease and salt-wasting conditions.

Q4. Drug given antenatally to enhance fetal lung maturity?
Betamethasone
Crosses placenta effectively.

Q5. Glucocorticoid that does not cross placenta?
Prednisolone
Inactivated by placental enzymes.

Q6. Drug used in overnight dexamethasone suppression test?
Dexamethasone
Screens for Cushing's syndrome.

Q7. Inhibitor of steroid synthesis used in Cushing's syndrome?
Ketoconazole
Inhibits 17,20-lyase and 11β-hydroxylase.

Q8. Adrenal enzyme blocked by metyrapone?
11β-hydroxylase
Causes buildup of 11-deoxycortisol.

Q9. Common side effect of long-term glucocorticoids?
Osteoporosis
Also hyperglycemia, infections, hypertension.

Q10. Most common endogenous glucocorticoid?
Cortisol
Follows diurnal rhythm.

Q11. Insulin type with rapid onset and short duration?
Insulin lispro
Given immediately before meals.

Q12. Long-acting basal insulin with no peak?
Insulin glargine
Mimics steady basal insulin.

Q13. Insulin used in diabetic ketoacidosis (DKA)?
Regular insulin (IV)
Short-acting and suitable for IV use.

Q14. Oral antidiabetic agent preferred in obese patients?
Metformin
Promotes weight neutrality or loss.

Q15. Metformin mechanism of action?
Inhibits hepatic gluconeogenesis
Also ↑ insulin sensitivity.

Q16. Major side effect of metformin?
Lactic acidosis
Especially in renal dysfunction.

Q17. Sulfonylurea mechanism?
Closes ATP-sensitive K^+ channels in β-cells
Stimulates insulin release.

Q18. Sulfonylurea with longest duration and highest hypoglycemia risk?
Glyburide (glibenclamide)
Avoid in elderly.

Q19. Rapid-acting insulin secretagogue?
Repaglinide
Similar action to sulfonylureas, but shorter duration.

Q20. Thiazolidinedione mechanism?
PPAR-γ activation
Increases insulin sensitivity.

Q21. TZD associated with weight gain and fluid retention?
Pioglitazone
Risk of heart failure exacerbation.

Q22. GLP-1 analog example?
Exenatide
Delays gastric emptying, ↑ satiety.

Q23. DPP-4 inhibitor example?
Sitagliptin
Increases endogenous GLP-1 levels.

Q24. Major benefit of GLP-1 agonists?
Weight loss
Low hypoglycemia risk when used alone.

Q25. SGLT2 inhibitor example?
Empagliflozin
Promotes glycosuria, lowers BP and weight.

Q26. Major adverse effect of SGLT2 inhibitors?
Genital infections
Due to glucosuria.

Q27. Alpha-glucosidase inhibitor mechanism?
Delays carbohydrate absorption
Reduces postprandial glucose.

Q28. Drug that lowers glucagon, slows gastric emptying?
Pramlintide (amylin analog)
Used in both T1DM and T2DM.

Q29. Hormone responsible for post-meal insulin spike?
GLP-1
Incretin effect.

Q30. Insulin effect on potassium?
Drives K^+ into cells
Used in hyperkalemia management.

Q31. Drug of choice for hyperprolactinemia?
Bromocriptine or Cabergoline
Dopamine agonists ↓ prolactin secretion.

Q32. Drug used in acromegaly to suppress GH?
Octreotide
Somatostatin analog, also used for variceal bleeding.

Q33. Pegvisomant mechanism?
GH receptor antagonist
Normalizes IGF-1 in acromegaly.

Q34. Somatostatin analog used in carcinoid syndrome?
Octreotide
Controls flushing and diarrhea.

Q35. Recombinant GH used in GH deficiency?
Somatropin
Promotes linear growth in children.

Q36. Drug used in nephrogenic diabetes insipidus?
Thiazide diuretics
Reduce polyuria via volume contraction.

Q37. DOC in central diabetes insipidus?
Desmopressin (DDAVP)
ADH analog with minimal vasoconstriction.

Q38. Drug causing nephrogenic diabetes insipidus?
Lithium
Interferes with ADH action in kidneys.

Q39. Thyroid hormone used in hypothyroidism?
Levothyroxine (T4)
Long half-life, converted to T3 peripherally.

Q40. Liothyronine is?
T3 hormone
Shorter acting, more potent.

Q41. Antithyroid drug safe in first trimester of pregnancy?
Propylthiouracil (PTU)
Inhibits thyroid hormone synthesis and peripheral T4→T3 conversion.

Q42. Antithyroid drug preferred in second and third trimesters?
Methimazole
Teratogenic in 1st trimester, safer later.

Q43. Antithyroid drug causing agranulocytosis?
Both PTU and methimazole
Monitor WBC count with sore throat/fever.

Q44. Drug used for rapid symptom relief in thyrotoxicosis?
Propranolol
Blocks β-adrenergic symptoms and inhibits peripheral T4→T3 conversion.

Q45. Radioactive iodine (I-131) is contraindicated in?
Pregnancy and lactation
Permanent hypothyroidism is a risk.

Q46. Lugol's iodine use before thyroid surgery?
Reduces vascularity of gland
Also acutely inhibits hormone release.

Q47. Thyroid storm acute management includes?
PTU + propranolol + steroids + iodine
Block synthesis, conversion, release, and symptoms.

Q48. Drug causing hypothyroidism as side effect?
Amiodarone
Contains iodine and inhibits deiodinase.

Q49. Drug used in hypercalcemia of malignancy?
Bisphosphonates (e.g., zoledronate)
Inhibit osteoclasts.

Q50. Calcitonin mechanism of action?
Inhibits osteoclast activity
Used short-term in hypercalcemia.

Q51. DOC for postmenopausal osteoporosis?
Bisphosphonates
↓ fracture risk.

Q52. Bisphosphonate administration instruction?
Take with water, remain upright 30 min
Prevent esophagitis.

Q53. Parathyroid hormone analog used for bone formation?
Teriparatide
Intermittent use → osteoblastic activity.

Q54. RANKL inhibitor used in osteoporosis?
Denosumab
Inhibits osteoclast formation.

Q55. Estrogen agonist–antagonist used in osteoporosis?
Raloxifene
Acts as estrogen in bone, anti-estrogen in breast.

Q56. Drug used for hypocalcemia in CKD?
Calcitriol
Active form of vitamin D.

Q57. Vitamin D analog causing less hypercalcemia?
Paricalcitol
Used in secondary hyperparathyroidism.

Q58. Cinacalcet mechanism?
Sensitizes calcium-sensing receptor
↓ PTH in secondary hyperparathyroidism.

Q59. Drug used in Paget's disease of bone?
Bisphosphonates
Suppress bone turnover.

Q60. Hormone increasing serum calcium and phosphate?
PTH
Increases resorption from bone, reabsorption of Ca^{2+}, excretion of phosphate.

Q61. Hormone that increases calcium but decreases phosphate?
Parathyroid hormone (PTH)
Increases renal phosphate excretion.

Q62. Hormone that decreases both calcium and phosphate?
Calcitonin
Inhibits bone resorption.

Q63. Vitamin D increases absorption of?
Both calcium and phosphate
Enhances intestinal absorption.

Q64. Hypocalcemia with high PTH suggests?
Vitamin D deficiency
Or PTH resistance (pseudohypoparathyroidism).

Q65. Hypocalcemia with low PTH suggests?
Hypoparathyroidism
Surgical or autoimmune cause.

Q66. Rapidly acting hypoglycemic agent (oral)?
Repaglinide
Short onset, used pre-meal.

Q67. Antidiabetic that delays gastric emptying?
Exenatide (GLP-1 analog)
Helps weight loss too.

Q68. Oral drug causing genital fungal infections?
SGLT2 inhibitors (e.g., dapagliflozin)
Due to glycosuria.

Q69. Drug that lowers postprandial glucose without causing hypoglycemia?
Acarbose
Delays carbohydrate absorption.

Q70. Insulin analog with ultra-long duration?
Insulin degludec
Duration > 24 hours.

Q71. Antidiabetic causing bladder cancer (rare concern)?
Pioglitazone
Controversial, but used cautiously.

Q72. Diabetes drug with cardiovascular mortality benefit?
Empagliflozin (SGLT2 inhibitor)
Also helps in heart failure.

Q73. Antidiabetic approved for weight loss?
Liraglutide (GLP-1 analog)
Approved for obesity with/without diabetes.

Q74. Drug class contraindicated in medullary thyroid cancer?
GLP-1 receptor agonists
Rodent studies → C-cell hyperplasia.

Q75. Antidiabetic that improves HDL levels?
Pioglitazone
Favourable lipid profile.

Q76. TSH suppression in thyroid cancer uses which drug?
Levothyroxine (T4)
Suppresses endogenous TSH to reduce tumor growth.

Q77. Anti-thyroid drug safe in thyroid storm?
Propylthiouracil (PTU)
Also blocks peripheral T4 to T3 conversion.

Q78. Drug that reduces thyroid hormone release acutely?
Iodine (Lugol's solution)
Used for pre-op preparation and thyroid storm.

Q79. Bone-forming drug used for limited duration only?
Teriparatide
Max 2 years use due to risk of osteosarcoma.

Q80. Calcimimetic used in CKD with high PTH?
Cinacalcet
Increases calcium receptor sensitivity.

Q81. Glucocorticoid used in congenital adrenal hyperplasia?
Hydrocortisone
Replaces cortisol and suppresses ACTH.

Q82. Antiandrogen used in prostate cancer?
Flutamide
Blocks androgen receptors.

Q83. Aromatase inhibitor example?
Anastrozole
Used in estrogen receptor–positive breast cancer.

Q84. GnRH analog used continuously for cancer therapy?
Leuprolide
Initially ↑ LH/FSH → then suppression.

Q85. Drug causing pseudohypoparathyroidism phenotype?
Albright hereditary osteodystrophy
Gs protein defect → PTH resistance.

Q86. Estrogen antagonist in breast but agonist in bone?
Raloxifene
Used in osteoporosis and breast cancer prevention.

Q87. Adverse effect of bisphosphonates on jaw?
Osteonecrosis of the jaw
Seen after dental procedures.

Q88. Estrogen therapy increases risk of?
Endometrial hyperplasia/cancer
Unopposed estrogen is risky.

Q89. Drug used in male-to-female hormone therapy?
Estradiol + spironolactone
Feminizing + antiandrogen effect.

Q90. Hormonal drug for emergency contraception?
Levonorgestrel
High-dose progestin.

Q91. Antidiabetic with risk of pancreatitis?
GLP-1 receptor agonists (e.g., exenatide)
Rare but serious adverse effect.

Q92. Drug causing disulfiram-like reaction with alcohol?
Chlorpropamide
1st gen sulfonylurea; also causes SIADH.

Q93. Antidiabetic drug safe in pregnancy?
Insulin
Does not cross placenta.

Q94. Drug used in insulinoma diagnosis?
Diazoxide
Opens K^+ channels, inhibits insulin release.

Q95. Long-acting GnRH analog causing initial flare?
Leuprolide
Used continuously in prostate cancer, endometriosis.

Q96. Somatostatin analog used in VIPoma?
Octreotide
Controls secretory diarrhea.

Q97. Drug that mimics TSH action in thyroid cancer scans?
Recombinant human TSH (rhTSH)
Stimulates iodine uptake.

Q98. Hormone with opposite action to insulin?
Glucagon
Increases glycogenolysis, gluconeogenesis.

Q99. Glucagon used clinically in?
Beta-blocker overdose
Increases cAMP via Gs pathway.

Q100. Oral antidiabetic causing megaloblastic anemia?
Metformin (rarely)
Via B12 malabsorption in long-term use.

Q101. Drug that increases insulin sensitivity in muscles and fat?
Pioglitazone
Acts via PPAR-γ receptor.

Q102. Hypercalcemia + suppressed PTH suggests?
Malignancy (PTHrP)
Rule out multiple myeloma or solid tumors.

Q103. Bisphosphonate used IV for severe hypercalcemia?
Zoledronate
Also used in bone metastases.

Q104. Drug used for prevention of chemotherapy-induced bone loss?
Denosumab
RANKL inhibitor.

Q105. Vitamin D analog safe in CKD?
Calcitriol
Active form; bypasses renal activation.

Q106. Hormone with catabolic effects on bone?
PTH (continuous exposure)
Intermittent exposure is anabolic.

Q107. Antiestrogen used in ovulation induction?
Clomiphene
Blocks estrogen feedback → ↑ FSH, LH.

Q108. Progestin used to delay periods?
Norethisterone
Taken for 5–7 days prior.

Q109. Hormonal contraceptive action on cervical mucus?
Progestins thicken it
Prevent sperm penetration.

Q110. Hormone that enhances Na^+ retention and K^+ loss?
Aldosterone
Acts on collecting duct.

Q111. Drug that antagonizes aldosterone receptor?
Spironolactone
Also antiandrogenic.

Q112. Spironolactone causes gynecomastia due to?
Antiandrogen effect
Also blocks testosterone synthesis.

Q113. Estrogen's effect on hepatic proteins?
Increases SHBG, clotting factors
Risk of thromboembolism.

Q114. Emergency contraceptive effective up to 5 days?
Ulipristal
Selective progesterone receptor modulator.

Q115. Drug used in medical abortion with misoprostol?
Mifepristone
Progesterone receptor antagonist.

Q116. Oxytocin used clinically for?
Inducing labor, controlling postpartum hemorrhage
Promotes uterine contractions.

Q117. Drug delaying preterm labor (tocolytic)?
Nifedipine
CCB → relaxes uterine smooth muscle.

Q118. DOC for prolactinoma?
Cabergoline
More selective and longer-acting than bromocriptine.

Q119. 21-hydroxylase deficiency treatment?
Hydrocortisone + fludrocortisone
Replaces deficient hormones and suppresses ACTH.

Q120. Hormone responsible for milk ejection reflex?
Oxytocin
Released in response to nipple stimulation.

Q1. Mechanism of action of penicillin?
Inhibits bacterial cell wall synthesis
Binds to penicillin-binding proteins (PBPs).

Q2. Bacterial enzyme that deactivates penicillin?
β-lactamase
Hydrolyzes the β-lactam ring.

Q3. Penicillinase-resistant penicillin?
Methicillin, nafcillin
Used in MSSA infections.

Q4. Extended-spectrum penicillin?
Amoxicillin
Covers H. influenzae, E. coli, Listeria, etc.

Q5. Amoxicillin is commonly combined with?
Clavulanic acid
β-lactamase inhibitor.

Q6. Antipseudomonal penicillins?
Piperacillin, ticarcillin
Often combined with tazobactam.

Q7. Cephalosporins are ineffective against?
Listeria, atypicals, MRSA (except 5th gen), Enterococci
"LAME" organisms.

Q8. 3rd generation cephalosporin for meningitis?
Ceftriaxone
Crosses blood–brain barrier well.

Q9. Cephalosporin for pseudomonas?
Ceftazidime (3rd gen), cefepime (4th gen)
Broad Gram-negative coverage.

Q10. Only cephalosporin active against MRSA?
Ceftaroline (5th gen)
Also binds altered PBPs.

Q11. Drug causing "red man syndrome"?
Vancomycin
Rapid infusion causes histamine release.

Q12. Vancomycin mechanism of action?
Inhibits cell wall synthesis by binding D-Ala-D-Ala
Bactericidal for Gram-positive bacteria.

Q13. Drug of choice for MRSA?
Vancomycin
Also linezolid and daptomycin.

Q14. Macrolide mechanism?
Inhibits 50S ribosomal subunit
Blocks translocation (bacteriostatic).

Q15. Macrolide with least drug interactions?
Azithromycin
Minimal CYP450 inhibition.

Q16. Tetracycline mechanism?
Binds 30S ribosomal subunit
Prevents tRNA attachment.

Q17. Tetracyclines are contraindicated in?
Pregnancy and children
Cause teeth discoloration, bone growth inhibition.

Q18. Tigecycline is useful against?
MDR bacteria including MRSA and VRE
Not used for bloodstream infections.

Q19. Aminoglycoside mechanism?
Binds 30S ribosomal subunit
Causes misreading of mRNA (bactericidal).

Q20. Major side effects of aminoglycosides?
Nephrotoxicity and ototoxicity
Avoid with loop diuretics or vancomycin.

Q21. Fluoroquinolone mechanism?
Inhibits DNA gyrase (topoisomerase II) and IV
Bactericidal for Gram-negatives.

Q22. Fluoroquinolone contraindication in children?
Cartilage damage, tendon rupture
Also avoided in pregnancy.

Q23. Antifolate combination used for UTI?
Trimethoprim + sulfamethoxazole (TMP-SMX)
Sequential blockade of folate synthesis.

Q24. TMP-SMX side effects?
Hyperkalemia, megaloblastic anemia, rash
Caution in renal dysfunction.

Q25. Sulfa drug allergy may cause?
Stevens–Johnson syndrome
Also hemolysis in G6PD deficiency.

Q26. Metronidazole mechanism?
Forms free radicals → DNA damage
Effective against anaerobes and protozoa.

Q27. Drug of choice for Clostridioides difficile?
Oral vancomycin or fidaxomicin
Metronidazole is second-line.

Q28. Drug causing disulfiram-like reaction with alcohol?
Metronidazole
Inhibits aldehyde dehydrogenase.

Q29. Linezolid major toxicity?
Bone marrow suppression, serotonin syndrome
Especially with SSRIs.

Q30. Daptomycin is inactivated by?
Pulmonary surfactant
Not used for pneumonia.

Q31. Daptomycin mechanism of action?
Disrupts bacterial cell membrane via depolarization
Bactericidal for Gram-positive organisms.

Q32. Antimicrobial causing eosinophilic pneumonia?
Daptomycin
Rare but serious complication.

Q33. Drug used in meningococcal prophylaxis?
Rifampin
Also active against TB.

Q34. Rifampin mechanism?
Inhibits DNA-dependent RNA polymerase
Prevents transcription.

Q35. Rifampin major adverse effect?
Orange discoloration of body fluids
Also hepatotoxicity.

Q36. Antitubercular drug causing optic neuritis?
Ethambutol
Causes red-green color blindness.

Q37. Ethambutol mechanism?
Inhibits arabinosyl transferase
Disrupts mycobacterial cell wall.

Q38. Isoniazid side effect reversed by pyridoxine?
Peripheral neuropathy
Due to B6 deficiency.

Q39. Isoniazid mechanism?
Inhibits mycolic acid synthesis
Prodrug activated by KatG enzyme.

Q40. Drug causing tubulointerstitial nephritis and Fanconi syndrome?
Tenofovir
Antiviral (nucleotide reverse transcriptase inhibitor).

Q41. First-line treatment for latent TB?
Isoniazid monotherapy
Usually for 6–9 months.

Q42. Drug used for leprosy causing skin pigmentation?
Clofazimine
Turns skin reddish-brown.

Q43. DOC for pneumocystis pneumonia (PCP)?
TMP-SMX
Also used for prophylaxis in HIV.

Q44. Drug for MAC prophylaxis in HIV?
Azithromycin
Given when CD4 <50.

Q45. DOC for toxoplasmosis prophylaxis in HIV?
TMP-SMX
CD4 count <100.

Q46. DOC for Toxoplasma gondii encephalitis?
Pyrimethamine + sulfadiazine + leucovorin
Leucovorin prevents folate deficiency.

Q47. Drug causing tendon rupture and QT prolongation?
Fluoroquinolones
Avoid with other QT-prolonging drugs.

Q48. Oral anaerobic coverage: above diaphragm vs below?
Clindamycin (above), Metronidazole (below)
Divides GI and respiratory anaerobes.

Q49. Drug of choice for Babesia infection?
Atovaquone + azithromycin
Malaria-like protozoal infection.

Q50. Antifungal inhibiting ergosterol synthesis?
Azoles (e.g., fluconazole)
Inhibit 14-α-demethylase.

Q51. Amphotericin B mechanism?
Binds ergosterol → forms membrane pores
Broad-spectrum fungicidal.

Q52. Major toxicity of amphotericin B?
Nephrotoxicity
Also causes hypokalemia, hypomagnesemia.

Q53. Echinocandin antifungals target?
β-glucan synthesis in fungal cell wall
Drugs: caspofungin, micafungin.

Q54. Drug used for cryptococcal meningitis?
Amphotericin B + flucytosine
Synergistic combination.

Q55. Flucytosine mechanism of action?
Inhibits fungal DNA and RNA synthesis
Converted to 5-FU inside fungal cells.

Q56. Antifungal causing gynecomastia?
Ketoconazole
Inhibits steroid synthesis.

Q57. Drug used for oral candidiasis (thrush)?
Nystatin (topical)
Not absorbed systemically.

Q58. Azole used in Aspergillus treatment?
Voriconazole
First-line for invasive aspergillosis.

Q59. First-line antifungal in neutropenic fever?
Caspofungin
Covers Candida and Aspergillus.

Q60. Drug of choice for invasive mucormycosis?
Liposomal amphotericin B
Voriconazole is ineffective.

Q61. Drug of choice for dermatophytosis (tinea infection)?
Terbinafine
Inhibits squalene epoxidase.

Q62. Antifungal used in onychomycosis?
Terbinafine
Long treatment course for nail infections.

Q63. Griseofulvin mechanism of action?
Disrupts fungal mitosis by binding microtubules
Deposits in keratin.

Q64. Antifungal inducing cytochrome P450 enzymes?
Griseofulvin
Reduces effectiveness of oral contraceptives.

Q65. Drug used in acyclovir-resistant HSV?
Foscarnet
Inhibits viral DNA polymerase directly.

Q66. Foscarnet side effect?
Hypocalcemia, seizures
Chelates divalent cations.

Q67. Acyclovir mechanism?
Guanosine analog, inhibits viral DNA polymerase
Activated by viral thymidine kinase.

Q68. Valacyclovir is a prodrug of?
Acyclovir
Better oral bioavailability.

Q69. DOC for CMV retinitis in immunocompromised?
Ganciclovir
Bone marrow suppression is major toxicity.

Q70. Drug used for CMV resistant to ganciclovir?
Foscarnet or cidofovir
No activation by viral kinase required.

Q71. Antiviral safe in pregnancy for influenza?
Oseltamivir
Neuraminidase inhibitor.

Q72. Amantadine mechanism?
Inhibits M2 proton channel in influenza A
No longer recommended due to resistance.

Q73. Antiretroviral causing hyperpigmentation of palms/soles?
Emtricitabine
NRTI class.

Q74. Zidovudine major adverse effect?
Bone marrow suppression
Used in vertical transmission prevention.

Q75. Tenofovir side effect?
Fanconi syndrome, renal toxicity
Especially with long-term use.

Q76. NNRTI causing vivid dreams and CNS side effects?
Efavirenz
Also teratogenic.

Q77. Protease inhibitor causing lipodystrophy?
Indinavir
Also causes nephrolithiasis.

Q78. HIV drug class causing hepatotoxicity and hyperglycemia?
Protease inhibitors
Ritonavir-boosted drugs especially.

Q79. HIV entry inhibitor binding CCR5?
Maraviroc
Tropism testing required before use.

Q80. HIV fusion inhibitor?
Enfuvirtide
Binds gp41 to prevent fusion.

Q81. Integrase inhibitor used in ART?
Dolutegravir
Blocks viral DNA integration into host genome.

Q82. Dolutegravir contraindicated in?
Early pregnancy
Risk of neural tube defects.

Q83. First-line ART regimen includes which classes?
2 NRTIs + 1 integrase inhibitor
Preferred for efficacy and safety.

Q84. Antihelminthic inhibiting microtubule synthesis?
Albendazole
Effective against roundworms, tapeworms.

Q85. DOC for neurocysticercosis?
Albendazole + steroids
Controls inflammation due to dying cysts.

Q86. Mebendazole vs albendazole: difference?
Albendazole has better tissue penetration
Preferred in systemic infections.

Q87. DOC for filariasis (Wuchereria bancrofti)?
Diethylcarbamazine (DEC)
Kills microfilariae and adults.

Q88. Antihelminthic contraindicated in ocular cysticercosis?
Albendazole
Killing cysts may cause severe inflammation.

Q89. Ivermectin mechanism of action?
Enhances GABA transmission in parasites
DOC for onchocerciasis.

Q90. Drug causing Mazzotti reaction in onchocerciasis?
Ivermectin
Fever, rash, hypotension due to immune reaction.

Q91. Antimalarial used for radical cure of vivax/ovale malaria?
Primaquine
Kills liver hypnozoites.

Q92. Primaquine contraindicated in?
G6PD deficiency
Causes hemolysis.

Q93. Drug of choice for severe falciparum malaria?
IV artesunate
Rapid parasite clearance.

Q94. Oral antimalarial for chloroquine-resistant falciparum?
Artemether-lumefantrine
ACT (Artemisinin Combination Therapy).

Q95. Chloroquine mechanism of action?
Inhibits heme polymerization
Leads to toxic heme accumulation.

Q96. Antimalarial causing cinchonism?
Quinine
Includes tinnitus, headache, nausea.

Q97. Antimalarial causing hemolysis in G6PD patients?
Primaquine and quinine
Dose adjustment or avoidance needed.

Q98. Drug for leishmaniasis (kala-azar)?
Liposomal amphotericin B
Most effective and safe.

Q99. Oral drug for cutaneous leishmaniasis?
Miltefosine
Teratogenic; not for pregnant women.

Q100. DOC for trypanosomiasis (Chagas disease)?
Nifurtimox or benznidazole
Effective in acute phase.

Q101. Drug used for giardiasis and amoebiasis?
Metronidazole
Followed by luminal agent (e.g., paromomycin).

Q102. Drug used for asymptomatic intestinal amoebiasis?
Paromomycin
Non-absorbable luminal amebicide.

Q103. Anthelmintic causing spastic paralysis of helminths?
Pyrantel pamoate
Used for hookworms, roundworms.

Q104. Broad-spectrum anti-parasitic used in strongyloides and onchocerciasis?
Ivermectin
Single-dose oral therapy.

Q105. Drug used in schistosomiasis?
Praziquantel
Increases calcium permeability → worm paralysis.

Q106. Antiviral with nephrotoxicity potentiated by IV contrast?
Acyclovir
Adequate hydration reduces risk.

Q107. Antimicrobial safe in pregnancy for UTI?
Nitrofurantoin (except near term)
Avoid in G6PD deficiency.

Q108. Antifungal used in systemic candidiasis and cryptococcus?
Fluconazole
Good CSF penetration.

Q109. Tetracycline with best oral absorption?
Doxycycline
Also safe in renal failure.

Q110. Antibiotic contraindicated with milk and antacids?
Tetracyclines
Chelates with calcium, iron.

Q111. Drug causing gray baby syndrome?
Chloramphenicol
Due to immature glucuronidation in neonates.

Q112. Antibiotic causing aplastic anemia?
Chloramphenicol
Rare, but fatal idiosyncratic reaction.

Q113. Antibiotic class causing photosensitivity?
Tetracyclines and fluoroquinolones
Advise sun protection.

Q114. Antitubercular drug needing pyridoxine supplementation?
Isoniazid
Prevents neuropathy.

Q115. Macrolide used in atypical pneumonia?
Azithromycin
Covers Mycoplasma and Chlamydia.

Q116. Drug of choice for plague (Yersinia pestis)?
Streptomycin
An aminoglycoside.

Q117. DOC for actinomycosis?
Penicillin G
Long-duration therapy required.

Q118. DOC for nocardiosis?
TMP-SMX
Sulfa-sensitive aerobic filamentous bacteria.

Q119. Antibiotic for MRSA skin infections (oral)?
Linezolid or doxycycline
Also clindamycin, depending on resistance.

Q120. Best empirical coverage for sepsis in neutropenic patients?
Cefepime or meropenem
Broad-spectrum with pseudomonal coverage.

Q121. DOC for Brucellosis?
Doxycycline + rifampin
Dual therapy for ≥6 weeks.

Q122. DOC for tularemia?
Streptomycin
Francisella tularensis infection.

Q123. DOC for anthrax (inhalational)?
Ciprofloxacin + doxycycline
With antitoxin support.

Q124. DOC for syphilis (primary, secondary, latent)?
Benzathine penicillin G
Single IM dose for early stages.

Q125. Treatment for neurosyphilis?
IV penicillin G
High doses needed for CSF penetration.

Q126. DOC for gonorrhea?
Ceftriaxone IM
Often with azithromycin for chlamydia co-infection.

Q127. DOC for chlamydia (non-pregnant)?
Doxycycline
Azithromycin is single-dose alternative.

Q128. Chlamydia treatment in pregnancy?
Azithromycin
Doxycycline contraindicated.

Q129. DOC for bacterial vaginosis?
Metronidazole
Covers anaerobic Gardnerella.

Q130. Drug of choice for typhoid fever?
Ceftriaxone (in India), azithromycin
Fluoroquinolones losing efficacy.

Q131. DOC for enteric fever in carriers?
Ciprofloxacin
Eradicates chronic gallbladder carriage.

Q132. DOC for cholera?
Doxycycline (single dose)
ORS remains most important.

Q133. DOC for traveler's diarrhea (ETEC)?
Azithromycin or ciprofloxacin
Also loperamide + hydration.

Q134. DOC for bacterial endocarditis prophylaxis (dental)?
Amoxicillin
In patients with valvular disease.

Q135. Empirical therapy for infective endocarditis?
Vancomycin + gentamicin
Until culture report available.

Q136. Drug of choice for Listeria meningitis?
Ampicillin
Especially in neonates, elderly.

Q137. Drug of choice for tetanus?
Metronidazole
Plus antitoxin, sedation, and supportive care.

Q138. DOC for diphtheria?
Erythromycin or penicillin
Plus diphtheria antitoxin.

Q139. DOC for pertussis?
Azithromycin
Also used for post-exposure prophylaxis.

Q140. Antibiotic for early Lyme disease?
Doxycycline
Amoxicillin in children or pregnancy.

Q141. DOC for late-stage Lyme or carditis?
Ceftriaxone
IV route preferred.

Q142. DOC for Mycoplasma pneumoniae?
Azithromycin or doxycycline
No cell wall, so β-lactams ineffective.

Q143. DOC for Legionella pneumonia?
Azithromycin or levofloxacin
Needs intracellular penetration.

Q144. Antibiotic that causes serotonin syndrome with SSRIs?
Linezolid
Monitor for hyperreflexia, agitation.

Q145. Best oral antibiotic for anaerobes above diaphragm?
Clindamycin
Risk of C. diff infection.

Q146. Drug of choice for actinomyces infections?
Penicillin G
Long-term therapy required.

Q147. DOC for nocardia (brain abscess)?
TMP-SMX
Sulfonamide-sensitive filamentous bacteria.

Q148. Drug used for prophylaxis after dog bite?
Amoxicillin-clavulanate
Covers Pasteurella and anaerobes.

Q149. Antimicrobial for human bite wound?
Amoxicillin-clavulanate
Also for clenched-fist injuries.

Q150. DOC for cat scratch disease?
Azithromycin
Bartonella henselae infection.

Q151. DOC for Haemophilus influenzae (non-β-lactamase strain)?
Amoxicillin
If resistant, use augmentin or 3rd gen cephalosporin.

Q152. Antibiotic combination causing nephrotoxicity?
Vancomycin + aminoglycoside
Monitor creatinine.

Q153. DOC for pseudomembranous colitis (C. difficile)?
Oral vancomycin
Fidaxomicin is alternative.

Q154. Bacteriostatic protein synthesis inhibitors?
Tetracyclines, macrolides, chloramphenicol
Reversible inhibition of ribosomes.

Q155. Bactericidal protein synthesis inhibitors?
Aminoglycosides
Irreversible ribosome inhibition.

Q156. Beta-lactam with activity against Pseudomonas?
Piperacillin + tazobactam
Also cefepime, meropenem.

Q157. DOC for epiglottitis (H. influenzae)?
Ceftriaxone
Also covers other URTI pathogens.

Q158. Drug causing lupus-like syndrome?
Isoniazid
Slow acetylators at higher risk.

Q159. Prophylaxis against bacterial endocarditis in penicillin allergy?
Clindamycin or azithromycin
Alternative to amoxicillin.

Q160. Drug for malaria prophylaxis in chloroquine-resistant areas?
Mefloquine or doxycycline
Weekly or daily regimen.

Q161. Mefloquine adverse effect?
Neuropsychiatric symptoms
Avoid in mental health disorders.

Q162. Antibiotic that inhibits bacterial transpeptidase?
Penicillins and cephalosporins
Block cell wall cross-linking.

Q163. Linezolid mechanism of action?
Inhibits 50S initiation complex
Prevents protein synthesis initiation.

Q164. Drug of choice for VRE (vancomycin-resistant enterococcus)?
Linezolid or daptomycin
Based on infection site.

Q165. Macrolide used for MAC prophylaxis?
Azithromycin
CD4 count <50.

Q166. Antibiotic safe in pregnancy and renal failure?
Azithromycin
No nephrotoxicity or teratogenicity.

Q167. DOC for aspiration pneumonia (anaerobes)?
Clindamycin
Covers anaerobes from oral flora.

Q168. Drug contraindicated in myasthenia gravis?
Aminoglycosides
Worsen neuromuscular transmission.

Q169. UTI prophylaxis in recurrent infections?
Nitrofurantoin (low-dose at night)
Long-term safety in females.

Q170. Antimicrobial with high post-antibiotic effect?
Aminoglycosides
Activity persists even after drug levels fall.

Q171. First-line anti-leprosy regimen?
Rifampin + dapsone + clofazimine
Multibacillary treatment.

Q172. Antitubercular drug safe in pregnancy?
Isoniazid
Supplement with pyridoxine.

Q173. DOC for bacterial meningitis in adults?
Ceftriaxone + vancomycin
Add ampicillin if Listeria suspected.

Q174. Drug for Helicobacter pylori eradication?
PPI + clarithromycin + amoxicillin/metronidazole
Triple or quadruple therapy.

Q175. Anti-TB drug with hepatotoxicity risk?
Isoniazid > rifampin > pyrazinamide
Monitor LFTs.

Q176. Antimicrobial with post-exposure prophylaxis for meningitis?
Rifampin
Alternative: ciprofloxacin or ceftriaxone.

Q177. DOC for pertussis prophylaxis?
Azithromycin
For close contacts.

Q178. Antiviral safe in renal failure?
Acyclovir (dose adjustment needed)
Hydration essential.

Q179. Drug of choice for enterococcal endocarditis?
Ampicillin + gentamicin
Synergistic killing.

Q180. Antimicrobial causing QT prolongation?
Macrolides, fluoroquinolones, azoles
Avoid with other QT drugs.

Q181. Drug that covers both MRSA and Pseudomonas?
Ceftaroline (MRSA) + ceftazidime-avibactam (Pseudomonas)
No single agent covers both fully.

Q182. Antibiotic contraindicated with SSRIs?
Linezolid
Risk of serotonin syndrome.

Q183. Drug used for typhus (Rickettsia)?
Doxycycline
Even in children when life-threatening.

Q184. Antibiotic for plague prophylaxis (post-exposure)?
Doxycycline or ciprofloxacin
7-day course.

Q185. Antibiotic for trench fever (Bartonella quintana)?
Doxycycline + gentamicin
Often in homeless/immunosuppressed.

Q186. DOC for resistant Acinetobacter infections?
Colistin
Last-resort, nephrotoxic.

Q187. Antibiotic inhibiting dihydropteroate synthase?
Sulfonamides
First step in folate pathway.

Q188. Antibiotic inhibiting dihydrofolate reductase?
Trimethoprim
Second step in folate pathway.

Q189. Antibiotic for Yersinia enterocolitica?
Doxycycline
For systemic disease.

Q190. Broadest spectrum β-lactam?
Carbapenems (e.g., meropenem)
Resistant to most β-lactamases.

Q191. Drug of choice for prosthetic valve endocarditis?
Vancomycin + gentamicin + rifampin
Covers biofilm and MRSA.

Q192. Beta-lactamase inhibitor with sulbactam?
Ampicillin
Effective in β-lactamase producers.

Q193. Anti-leprosy drug causing red-black skin discoloration?
Clofazimine
Lipophilic and tissue-binding.

Q194. DOC for Q fever (Coxiella burnetii)?
Doxycycline
Intracellular pathogen.

Q195. Lincosamide antibiotic?
Clindamycin
Protein synthesis inhibitor.

Q196. Fluoroquinolone active against anaerobes?
Moxifloxacin
Not reliable against Pseudomonas.

Q197. Antibiotic inhibiting topoisomerase IV?
Fluoroquinolones
Also inhibit DNA gyrase.

Q198. Drug causing pseudotumor cerebri?
Tetracyclines
Increased intracranial pressure.

Q199. Drug with dual antimalarial and anti-inflammatory use?

Hydroxychloroquine
Used in SLE, RA.

Q200. Antibiotic causing Achilles tendon rupture?

Fluoroquinolones
Especially in elderly or steroid use.

Autacoids & Anti-inflammatory Drugs

Q1. Autacoids are?
Locally acting chemical mediators
Include histamine, serotonin, prostaglandins, etc.

Q2. Histamine stored in?
Mast cells and basophils
Released during allergic reactions.

Q3. H1 receptor effects include?
Vasodilation, bronchoconstriction, itching
Involved in allergy and inflammation.

Q4. H2 receptor stimulation leads to?
Increased gastric acid secretion
Located on parietal cells of stomach.

Q5. First-generation H1 blockers cause sedation because?
Cross blood–brain barrier
Examples: diphenhydramine, chlorpheniramine.

Q6. Second-generation H1 blockers are less sedative because?
Poor CNS penetration
Examples: loratadine, cetirizine.

Q7. H1 blocker used in motion sickness?
Promethazine or dimenhydrinate
Anticholinergic and antihistaminic effects.

Q8. H1 blocker with antiemetic properties?
Meclizine
Used in vertigo and nausea.

Q9. DOC for anaphylaxis?
Epinephrine
Reverses bronchospasm and hypotension.

Q10. H2 blockers used for?
Peptic ulcers, GERD
Eg: ranitidine, famotidine.

Q11. Adverse effect of cimetidine?
Gynecomastia, CYP450 inhibition
Least used among H2 blockers.

Q12. 5-HT1 receptor agonist used in migraine?
Sumatriptan
Vasoconstriction of cerebral vessels.

Q13. Sumatriptan contraindicated in?
Coronary artery disease
Due to vasoconstrictive potential.

Q14. 5-HT3 receptor antagonist used in vomiting?
Ondansetron
Acts on CTZ and gut.

Q15. 5-HT2 antagonists used as antipsychotics?
Risperidone, olanzapine
Also block dopamine.

Q16. Serotonin syndrome is caused by?
Excess serotonergic activity
Often due to drug interactions.

Q17. DOC for serotonin syndrome?
Cyproheptadine
5-HT2 antagonist.

Q18. Prostaglandins derived from?
Arachidonic acid
Via COX pathway.

Q19. COX-1 enzyme function?
Maintains gastric mucosa, platelet function
Constitutive.

Q20. COX-2 enzyme function?
Induced in inflammation
Targeted by selective NSAIDs.

Q21. PG analog used for cervical ripening?
Misoprostol
PGE1 analog.

Q22. PG analog used for glaucoma?
Latanoprost
Increases aqueous outflow.

Q23. PG analog used to maintain PDA?
Alprostadil (PGE1)
Keeps ductus open.

Q24. NSAID that irreversibly inhibits COX?
Aspirin
Used for cardioprotection.

Q25. Low-dose aspirin inhibits?
Platelet aggregation (via TXA2)
Cardioprotective dose: 75–100 mg/day.

Q26. Aspirin contraindicated in children with viral illness?
Risk of Reye's syndrome
Encephalopathy + hepatic failure.

Q27. Selective COX-2 inhibitor?
Celecoxib
Less GI toxicity, but CV risk ↑.

Q28. NSAID safest in peptic ulcer patients?
Celecoxib
Avoids COX-1 inhibition.

Q29. NSAID safest in renal failure?
None ideally; if needed, use cautiously with monitoring.

Q30. NSAID causing closure of PDA?
Indomethacin
Also used in preterm infants.

Q31. NSAID commonly associated with tinnitus at high doses?
Aspirin
Sign of salicylate toxicity.

Q32. Acetaminophen mechanism of action?
Weak COX inhibitor in CNS
Analgesic and antipyretic, not anti-inflammatory.

Q33. Acetaminophen overdose causes?
Hepatotoxicity
Due to toxic metabolite NAPQI.

Q34. Antidote for acetaminophen toxicity?
N-acetylcysteine
Replenishes glutathione.

Q35. NSAID with high risk of gastrointestinal bleeding?
Piroxicam
Potent and long-acting.

Q36. NSAID safe in pregnancy (up to 32 weeks)?
Paracetamol
NSAIDs contraindicated in 3rd trimester.

Q37. NSAID causing pseudoporphyria in children?
Naproxen
Photodistributed skin lesions.

Q38. DMARD used in rheumatoid arthritis?
Methotrexate
First-line disease-modifying agent.

Q39. Methotrexate mechanism of action?
Inhibits dihydrofolate reductase
Decreases DNA synthesis.

Q40. Methotrexate toxicity prevented by?
Leucovorin (folinic acid) rescue
Prevents bone marrow suppression.

Q41. DMARD causing retinal toxicity?
Hydroxychloroquine
Regular eye exams needed.

Q42. Sulfasalazine used in?
RA, ulcerative colitis
Immunosuppressive and anti-inflammatory.

Q43. Anti-TNF agents used in RA?
Infliximab, etanercept, adalimumab
Target TNF-α cytokine.

Q44. Major side effect of anti-TNF therapy?
Reactivation of TB
Screen with Mantoux/IGRA before use.

Q45. Etanercept is a?
TNF receptor fusion protein
Acts as a decoy receptor.

Q46. Infliximab is a?
Monoclonal antibody against TNF-α
Given IV.

Q47. Janus kinase (JAK) inhibitor used in RA?
Tofacitinib
Oral DMARD.

Q48. Prostaglandin analog used in erectile dysfunction?
Alprostadil
PGE1 analog.

Q49. PGI_2 analog used in pulmonary hypertension?
Epoprostenol
Potent vasodilator and platelet inhibitor.

Q50. Montelukast is a?
Leukotriene receptor antagonist
Used in asthma and allergic rhinitis.

Q51. Zileuton mechanism?
5-lipoxygenase inhibitor
Blocks leukotriene synthesis.

Q52. Antihistamine safe in pregnancy?
Loratadine or cetirizine
Non-sedating and category B.

Q53. H1 blocker causing maximal sedation?
Diphenhydramine
First-generation antihistamine.

Q54. Ranitidine banned due to?
NDMA impurity
Potential carcinogen.

Q55. Longest acting second-generation antihistamine?
Fexofenadine
Minimal sedation.

Q56. Aspirin effect on uric acid?
Low dose ↑ uric acid, high dose ↓ uric acid
Not used in gout.

Q57. NSAID of choice in acute gout?
Indomethacin
Potent anti-inflammatory action.

Q58. Drug used for prevention of NSAID-induced ulcers?
Misoprostol
PGE1 analog; causes diarrhea and abortion.

Q59. DMARD with risk of hemolysis in G6PD deficiency?
Sulfasalazine
Monitor blood counts.

Q60. Biologic agent targeting IL-6 in RA?
Tocilizumab
Used in refractory RA cases.

Q61. Cytokine blocked by anakinra?
Interleukin-1 (IL-1)
Used in RA and periodic fever syndromes.

Q62. NSAID most commonly used for PDA closure in neonates?
Indomethacin
Promotes ductal constriction.

Q63. NSAID least likely to cause GI irritation?
Celecoxib
COX-2 selective.

Q64. Risk with COX-2 selective NSAIDs?
Cardiovascular thrombotic events
Due to imbalance between prostacyclin and thromboxane.

Q65. PG analog used to terminate early pregnancy?
Misoprostol
Usually with mifepristone.

Q66. NSAID with once-daily dosing?
Piroxicam
Long half-life.

Q67. Antihistamine used in insomnia?
Diphenhydramine
Common OTC sleep aid.

Q68. Antihistamine used in chemotherapy-induced nausea?
Promethazine
H1 blocker with anticholinergic effect.

Q69. Uricosuric drug increasing uric acid excretion?
Probenecid
Inhibits reabsorption in renal tubules.

Q70. Contraindication to probenecid?
History of uric acid stones
Risk of nephrolithiasis.

Q71. Anti-inflammatory effect of colchicine?
Inhibits microtubule polymerization
Prevents neutrophil chemotaxis.

Q72. First-line agent for acute gout if NSAIDs contraindicated?
Colchicine
Effective if given early.

Q73. Allopurinol mechanism?
Inhibits xanthine oxidase
Prevents uric acid formation.

Q74. Febuxostat vs. allopurinol?
Both inhibit xanthine oxidase
Febuxostat may be used in renal failure.

Q75. Drug causing severe skin rash (e.g., SJS) in HLA-B 5801 positive individuals?
Allopurinol
Screening recommended in some populations.

Q76. Drug interactions with allopurinol?
Increases toxicity of azathioprine, 6-MP
Xanthine oxidase metabolizes them.

Q77. IL-1 receptor antagonist used in autoinflammatory syndromes?
Anakinra
Less commonly used in RA.

Q78. NSAID with risk of pancreatitis?
Sulindac
Rare but reported.

Q79. PG analog used in impotence therapy?
Alprostadil
Intracavernosal injection or urethral insert.

Q80. PGF2α analog used in obstetrics?
Carboprost
Used to induce abortion or treat postpartum hemorrhage.

Q81. PG analog used for gastric protection in NSAID users?
Misoprostol
Causes abdominal cramps and diarrhea.

Q82. NSAID most associated with hepatotoxicity?
Diclofenac
Monitor liver enzymes with prolonged use.

Q83. NSAID used for closure of PDA, but not in India due to availability issues?
Ibuprofen IV
Safer than indomethacin in some studies.

Q84. Anti-histamine used in serotonin syndrome?
Cyproheptadine
Also has 5-HT2 blocking properties.

Q85. Drug causing nasal stuffiness via prostaglandin release?
Indomethacin
Seen in some patients.

Q86. PGI2 (prostacyclin) effects?
Vasodilation, inhibits platelet aggregation
Opposes thromboxane A2.

Q87. Drug used in pulmonary arterial hypertension (PAH)?
Epoprostenol
Short half-life, continuous IV infusion.

Q88. NSAID contraindicated in asthma with nasal polyps?
Aspirin
Risk of aspirin-exacerbated respiratory disease (AERD).

Q89. Leukotriene involved in bronchoconstriction?
LTC4, LTD4, LTE4
Blocked by montelukast.

Q90. Most potent bronchoconstrictor among leukotrienes?
LTD4
Targeted by leukotriene receptor antagonists.

Q91. Drug class of zileuton?
5-lipoxygenase inhibitor
Prevents synthesis of leukotrienes.

Q92. Major toxicity of zileuton?
Hepatotoxicity
Monitor liver enzymes regularly.

Q93. Drug of choice for aspirin-induced asthma?
Montelukast
Leukotriene receptor antagonist.

Q94. Misoprostol mechanism of action?
PGE1 analog – ↑ mucus, ↓ acid
Protects gastric mucosa.

Q95. Most selective COX-2 inhibitor in India?
Etoricoxib
Less GI toxicity, more CV risk.

Q96. NSAID avoided in late pregnancy?
All NSAIDs
Risk of premature ductus closure.

Q97. Antihistamine safe in elderly with BPH?
Loratadine
Minimal anticholinergic effect.

Q98. PG analog used in glaucoma causing iris pigmentation?
Latanoprost
PGF2α analog.

Q99. PG analog causing uterine contraction?
Carboprost
Used for postpartum hemorrhage.

Q100. PG analog used in erectile dysfunction?
Alprostadil
Increases cAMP → vasodilation.

Q101. Use of leukotriene inhibitors in aspirin-exacerbated respiratory disease?
Reduce bronchoconstriction
Montelukast improves symptoms.

Q102. H1 blocker causing prolonged QT interval?
Terfenadine (withdrawn)
Fexofenadine is safer alternative.

Q103. NSAID with highest risk of renal damage?
Indomethacin
Potent vasoconstrictor of renal vessels.

Q104. Prostaglandin involved in fever?
PGE2
Acts on hypothalamic thermoregulatory center.

Q105. Antipyretic action of paracetamol is due to?
Inhibition of PGE2 synthesis in CNS
Reduces hypothalamic set-point.

Q106. PG involved in labor initiation?
PGF2α and PGE2
Used for cervical ripening and abortion.

Q107. Adverse effect of montelukast in children?
Nightmares, behavioral changes
Monitor mood symptoms.

Q108. PG analog used for neonatal ductus arteriosus maintenance?
Alprostadil
Keeps ductus open in congenital heart disease.

Q109. H2 receptor blockers that inhibit CYP450?
Cimetidine
Affects warfarin, theophylline metabolism.

Q110. DOC for NSAID-induced peptic ulcer?
Proton pump inhibitors (PPIs)
Superior to H2 blockers.

Q111. NSAID with platelet-sparing effect?
Celecoxib
Does not inhibit thromboxane A2.

Q112. Uricosuric agent that prolongs penicillin action?
Probenecid
Inhibits renal tubular secretion.

Q113. NSAID with low GI side effect and long half-life?
Etodolac
Preferential COX-2 activity.

Q114. Drug used for prevention of altitude sickness?
Acetazolamide
Carbonic anhydrase inhibitor → mild acidosis.

Q115. Use of dexamethasone in chemotherapy?
Anti-emetic & edema control
Commonly combined with 5-HT3 blockers.

Q116. Prostaglandin involved in vasodilation of afferent arteriole?
PGE2
Maintains GFR in low perfusion states.

Q117. NSAID contraindicated in CABG surgery patients?
Celecoxib
↑ risk of thrombotic events.

Q118. NSAID that inhibits both COX and LOX?
Licofelone (under trial)
Dual inhibitor, still experimental.

Q119. Dual-action drug for OA: COX inhibition + cartilage protection?
Diacerein
Slow-acting in osteoarthritis.

Q120. Common adverse effect of misoprostol?
Diarrhea and abdominal cramping
Also contraindicated in pregnancy (unless for abortion).

Q121. COX-1 predominant location and role?
Stomach, platelets, kidneys – protective functions
Maintains mucosal integrity, renal blood flow, platelet function.

Q122. COX-2 predominant role?
Inflammation and pain
Inducible during injury or infection.

Q123. Inhibition of prostacyclin (PGI2) leads to?
Increased thrombotic risk
Seen with COX-2 inhibitors.

Q124. Leukotriene that promotes neutrophil chemotaxis?
LTB4
Pro-inflammatory.

Q125. DOC for systemic mastocytosis symptoms (flushing, urticaria)?
H1 + H2 blockers
Block both histamine receptor types.

Q126. DOC for chronic urticaria?
Second-generation antihistamines
Eg: fexofenadine, loratadine.

Q127. Misoprostol contraindicated in?
Pregnancy
Causes uterine contractions.

Q128. DOC for motion sickness in pilots?
Scopolamine patch
Anticholinergic, long-acting.

Q129. Anti-TNF agent with lowest immunogenicity?
Adalimumab
Fully human monoclonal antibody.

Q130. PG analog used for cervical softening before labor?
Dinoprostone
PGE2 analog.

Q131. Long-term NSAID use causes salt and water retention by?
Decreasing prostaglandin-mediated vasodilation
Leads to hypertension, edema.

Q132. Drug causing paradoxical bronchospasm in asthmatics?
Aspirin
AERD – due to leukotriene overproduction.

Q133. DOC for cold urticaria?
Non-sedating H1 blockers
Prevent histamine-mediated response.

Q134. Prostaglandin analog causing increased eyelash growth?
Latanoprost
Cosmetic use derived from glaucoma treatment.

Q135. Cysteinyl leukotriene receptor antagonists?
Montelukast, zafirlukast
Block LTC4, LTD4, LTE4 receptors.

Q136. Biologic used in severe eosinophilic asthma?
Mepolizumab
Anti–IL-5 monoclonal antibody.

Q137. Antihistamine used in food allergies?
Diphenhydramine (IV in anaphylaxis adjunct)
Not primary drug – use epinephrine first.

Q138. NSAID most selective for COX-1?
Ketorolac
Potent analgesic; short-term use only.

Q139. NSAID safe in hemophilia?
None – avoid all
Paracetamol preferred.

Q140. DOC for menstrual cramps (primary dysmenorrhea)?
Mefenamic acid
Reduces prostaglandins causing uterine contraction.

Q141. Gout drug that inhibits uric acid synthesis?
Allopurinol
Xanthine oxidase inhibitor.

Q142. Gout drug that increases uric acid excretion?
Probenecid
Uricosuric agent.

Q143. PGI2 role in platelets?
Inhibits aggregation
Opposes thromboxane A2.

Q144. Drug that reduces methotrexate clearance?
NSAIDs
Risk of toxicity due to renal competition.

Q145. Biologic targeting IL-17 in psoriasis/RA?
Secukinumab
IL-17A inhibitor.

Q146. DMARD associated with retinal toxicity?
Hydroxychloroquine
Screen with fundus exams.

Q147. Most common cause of drug-induced lupus?
Hydralazine > isoniazid > procainamide
HLA-DR4 associated.

Q148. Drug causing nasal congestion as a side effect?
Indomethacin
Prostaglandin imbalance in nasal mucosa.

Q149. Paracetamol toxicity due to?
NAPQI metabolite accumulation
Depletes glutathione → liver necrosis.

Q150. Reason for not combining aspirin and warfarin?
Increased bleeding risk
Dual antiplatelet + anticoagulant effect.

Q151. NSAID with highest risk of hypersensitivity reactions?
Ibuprofen
Especially in NSAID-exacerbated respiratory disease.

Q152. PG analog used in Raynaud's phenomenon?
Iloprost
Improves blood flow in digital arteries.

Q153. Anti-inflammatory drug that causes hyperkalemia?
NSAIDs
Inhibit renal prostaglandins → ↓ renin → ↓ aldosterone.

Q154. Glucocorticoid used in cerebral edema?
Dexamethasone
Reduces capillary permeability.

Q155. NSAID with the longest half-life?
Piroxicam
Once-daily dosing.

Q156. Mast cell stabilizer used in allergic rhinitis and asthma?
Cromolyn sodium
Prevents degranulation.

Q157. PG that induces vomiting in overdose cases?
None directly – ipecac used earlier (withdrawn).
Misoprostol causes nausea, but not for overdose use.

Q158. Best NSAID for closing PDA in neonates?
Indomethacin
Constricts ductus arteriosus.

Q159. PG analog used in male infants with duct-dependent cardiac lesions?
Alprostadil
Maintains ductal patency.

Q160. PG analog that promotes gastric mucus production?
Misoprostol
Cytoprotective effect.

Q161. Cytokine suppressed by methotrexate in RA?
TNF-α
Also reduces IL-1, IL-6.

Q162. RA drug contraindicated in liver disease and alcoholics?
Methotrexate
Hepatotoxicity risk ↑.

Q163. NSAID preferred in post-op pain (parenteral)?
Ketorolac
Potent analgesic; short-term only.

Q164. Reason for low-dose aspirin preference in CV disease?
Selective thromboxane A2 inhibition
Minimal prostacyclin inhibition.

Q165. Drug that reduces aspirin's cardioprotective effect when given concurrently?
Ibuprofen
Competes at COX-1 binding site.

Q166. DMARD preferred in early RA with minimal symptoms?
Hydroxychloroquine
Mild/moderate cases, especially in females.

Q167. Biologic that inhibits IL-12 and IL-23?
Ustekinumab
Used in psoriasis, IBD.

Q168. Antihistamine used in anxiety and sedation pre-op?
Hydroxyzine
Also has antiemetic properties.

Q169. PG analog contraindicated in asthmatics due to bronchospasm risk?
Carboprost
PGF2α analog → bronchoconstriction.

Q170. NSAID safe for CV patients with minimal GI risk?
Naproxen
Least thrombotic risk among traditional NSAIDs.

Q171. NSAID contraindicated with anticoagulants?
All NSAIDs
↑ GI bleeding risk with warfarin.

Q172. Agent used for chemoprevention in colorectal cancer?
Aspirin
Especially in FAP and Lynch syndrome.

Q173. Antihistamine with best anti-motion sickness property?
Promethazine
H1 + anticholinergic effects.

Q174. Antihistamine with least sedation?
Fexofenadine
2nd gen, non-CNS penetrating.

Q175. PG analog that causes pigmentation of iris?
Latanoprost
Reversible with discontinuation.

Q176. Drug causing flushing via prostaglandin-mediated vasodilation?
Niacin
PGD2-mediated → prevented by aspirin.

Q177. NSAID that may cause hematologic toxicity?
Phenylbutazone (withdrawn)
Causes aplastic anemia.

Q178. First-line treatment for chronic urticaria?
Second-generation H1 blockers
Eg: loratadine, cetirizine.

Q179. NSAID contraindicated in depression or bipolar disorder?
Indomethacin
Can cause mood disturbances.

Q180. DMARD with highest risk of tuberculosis reactivation?
Infliximab
Screen for latent TB before therapy.

Q181. DOC for prophylaxis of NSAID-induced peptic ulcer in high-risk patients?
Proton Pump Inhibitors (PPIs)
Eg: omeprazole.

Q182. Leukotriene receptor antagonist used in allergic rhinitis?
Montelukast
Also effective in asthma.

Q183. NSAID preferred in gout patients with CV disease?
Naproxen
Least CV risk among NSAIDs.

Q184. Use of montelukast in exercise-induced asthma?
Preventive before activity
Taken 2 hours prior to exercise.

Q185. DOC for preeclampsia prevention in high-risk pregnancies?
Low-dose aspirin
Started after 12 weeks gestation.

Q186. Biologic DMARD with longest half-life?
Adalimumab
SC dosing every 2–3 weeks.

Q187. NSAID with high risk of skin rashes, SJS?
Oxicam group (piroxicam, meloxicam)
Long half-life drugs.

Q188. COX inhibition effect on prostacyclin?
Decreased PGI_2 synthesis
Reduces vasodilation, ↑ thrombosis risk.

Q189. DMARD that reduces lymphocyte proliferation by inhibiting pyrimidine synthesis?
Leflunomide
Inhibits dihydroorotate dehydrogenase.

Q190. Antihistamine safe for long-term use in children?
Cetirizine
Second-gen, minimal sedation.

Q191. PG analog contraindicated in glaucoma patients with uveitis?
Latanoprost
May worsen inflammation.

Q192. NSAID with topical and systemic formulations for OA?
Diclofenac
Available as gel, patch, tablets.

Q193. PG analog used in PAH and delivered via inhalation?
Iloprost
Short half-life; frequent dosing.

Q194. Drug useful in aspirin-induced angioedema?
Montelukast
Reduces leukotriene-mediated inflammation.

Q195. Antihistamine with additional mast cell stabilizing activity?
Ketotifen
Used in allergic conjunctivitis.

Q196. NSAID that increases lithium levels?
Ibuprofen
↓ renal clearance of lithium.

Q197. Misoprostol is contraindicated in?
Women of childbearing age not on contraception
Risk of abortion, uterine rupture.

Q198. PG analog with longest duration in glaucoma?
Travoprost
Once-daily dosing.

Q199. COX enzyme responsible for fever and pain?
COX-2
Induced by cytokines during inflammation.

Q200. Drug that can counteract flushing caused by niacin?
Aspirin (30 minutes before)
Blocks prostaglandin-mediated vasodilation.

Chemotherapy of Neoplastic Diseases

Q1. Alkylating agents act during which cell cycle phase?
Non-specific (any phase)
Cross-link DNA → prevent replication.

Q2. Cyclophosphamide toxicity?
Hemorrhagic cystitis
Prevented with mesna.

Q3. Ifosfamide major toxicity?
Neurotoxicity and hemorrhagic cystitis
Also prevented by mesna.

Q4. Drug used to protect bladder from cyclophosphamide toxicity?
Mesna
Binds acrolein.

Q5. Alkylating agent causing pulmonary fibrosis?
Busulfan
Also causes hyperpigmentation.

Q6. Nitrosourea used in brain tumors?
Carmustine
Crosses BBB.

Q7. Drug used in CML targeting BCR-ABL tyrosine kinase?
Imatinib
First targeted therapy.

Q8. Antimetabolites act during which cell cycle phase?
S phase
Inhibit DNA synthesis.

Q9. Methotrexate inhibits?
Dihydrofolate reductase
Prevents dTMP formation.

Q10. Rescue agent for methotrexate toxicity?
Leucovorin (folinic acid)
Protects normal cells.

Q11. 5-Fluorouracil (5-FU) inhibits?
Thymidylate synthase
Requires activation.

Q12. 5-FU toxicity enhanced by?
Leucovorin
Increases 5-FU binding to thymidylate synthase.

Q13. Capecitabine is a prodrug of?
5-FU
Oral fluoropyrimidine.

Q14. Cytarabine used primarily in?
AML
Pyrimidine analog.

Q15. Cytarabine toxicity?
Cerebellar ataxia and myelosuppression
Especially in high doses.

Q16. Purine analog used in ALL?
6-mercaptopurine
Inactivated by xanthine oxidase.

Q17. 6-MP toxicity increased with?
Allopurinol
Requires dose reduction.

Q18. Cladribine used in?
Hairy cell leukemia
Purine analog resistant to ADA.

Q19. Hydroxyurea mechanism?
Inhibits ribonucleotide reductase
S-phase specific.

Q20. Hydroxyurea used in?
CML, sickle cell disease
Increases fetal hemoglobin.

Q21. Vinca alkaloids act in which phase?
M phase
Inhibit microtubule polymerization.

Q22. Vincristine dose-limiting toxicity?
Peripheral neuropathy
Minimal marrow suppression.

Q23. Vinblastine toxicity?
Myelosuppression
"Blasts bone marrow".

Q24. Taxanes (e.g., paclitaxel) mechanism?
Stabilize microtubules → inhibit depolymerization
Arrest in M phase.

Q25. Paclitaxel major side effect?
Neuropathy, hypersensitivity reactions
Premedicate with steroids, antihistamines.

Q26. Etoposide inhibits?
Topoisomerase II
Causes double-strand DNA breaks.

Q27. Topotecan inhibits?
Topoisomerase I
Used in ovarian and small-cell lung cancer.

Q28. Doxorubicin mechanism?
Free radical generation + Topo II inhibition
Anthracycline class.

Q29. Doxorubicin cardiotoxicity prevented by?
Dexrazoxane
Iron chelator.

Q30. Bleomycin toxicity?
Pulmonary fibrosis
Also causes skin changes.

Q31. Drug causing hand-foot syndrome?
Capecitabine, 5-FU
Palmar-plantar erythrodysesthesia.

Q32. Cisplatin toxicity?
Nephrotoxicity, ototoxicity, nausea
Prevent renal damage with hydration.

Q33. Carboplatin vs. cisplatin toxicity?
Less nephrotoxic, more myelosuppressive
Safer in renal failure.

Q34. Oxaliplatin key toxicity?
Cold-induced peripheral neuropathy
Common in colon cancer regimens.

Q35. Monoclonal antibody against HER2?
Trastuzumab
Used in HER2+ breast cancer.

Q36. Trastuzumab toxicity?
Cardiotoxicity
Monitor LVEF during therapy.

Q37. EGFR monoclonal antibody?
Cetuximab
Used in colorectal and head/neck cancers.

Q38. Cetuximab only works if?
KRAS wild type
Ineffective in KRAS mutations.

Q39. VEGF inhibitor monoclonal antibody?
Bevacizumab
Inhibits angiogenesis.

Q40. Bevacizumab side effect?
Hypertension, bleeding, delayed wound healing
Also proteinuria.

Q41. Rituximab targets?
CD20
Used in B-cell lymphomas, RA.

Q42. Rituximab major adverse effect?
Infusion reaction
Risk of reactivation of HBV.

Q43. Proteasome inhibitor in multiple myeloma?
Bortezomib
Causes peripheral neuropathy.

Q44. TKI targeting VEGF receptors?
Sunitinib, sorafenib
Used in RCC, GIST.

Q45. Drug causing hemorrhagic cystitis + neurotoxicity?
Ifosfamide
Always co-administer mesna.

Q46. Common side effect of TKIs like erlotinib?
Acneiform rash
Correlates with efficacy.

Q47. Drug used for tumor lysis syndrome prophylaxis?
Allopurinol
↓ uric acid.

Q48. Recombinant urate oxidase for tumor lysis?
Rasburicase
Converts uric acid to allantoin.

Q49. Growth factor used to reduce neutropenia in chemotherapy?
Filgrastim (G-CSF)
Stimulates neutrophil production.

Q50. Anticancer drug that enhances red cell production?
Epoetin alfa
Used in chemotherapy-induced anemia.

Q51. Drug used for AML induction therapy?
Cytarabine + daunorubicin ("7+3 regimen")
Standard induction protocol.

Q52. Common oral prodrug used in colon cancer?
Capecitabine
Converted to 5-FU in tumor tissues.

Q53. Platinum compound not causing nephrotoxicity?
Carboplatin
Preferred in renal compromise.

Q54. Chemotherapy agent causing SIADH?
Cyclophosphamide
Dose-dependent water retention.

Q55. Alkylating agent most associated with secondary leukemia?
Melphalan
Especially after long-term use.

Q56. Target of palbociclib in breast cancer?
CDK4/6
Prevents cell cycle progression.

Q57. Drug used in ER-positive breast cancer (postmenopausal)?
Letrozole
Aromatase inhibitor.

Q58. Tamoxifen mechanism?
SERM – Estrogen antagonist in breast
Agonist in endometrium, bone.

Q59. Tamoxifen side effect?
Endometrial carcinoma
Due to agonist effect.

Q60. Fulvestrant differs from tamoxifen by being a?
Pure estrogen receptor antagonist
No agonist action.

Q61. Chemotherapy agent that acts as androgen receptor blocker?
Flutamide
Used in prostate cancer.

Q62. GnRH analog used in prostate and breast cancer?
Leuprolide
Continuous use suppresses LH/FSH.

Q63. Drug causing hot flashes and impotence in men?
Leuprolide
Due to testosterone suppression.

Q64. Chemotherapeutic agent causing blue skin hyperpigmentation?
Busulfan
Also causes lung fibrosis.

Q65. Chemo drug that causes photosensitivity?
5-FU
Advise sun protection.

Q66. Drug causing jaw osteonecrosis?
Zoledronate (bisphosphonate)
Especially with dental procedures.

Q67. Drug that inhibits epigenetic modification via HDAC inhibition?
Vorinostat
Used in cutaneous T-cell lymphoma.

Q68. TKI used in renal cell carcinoma (RCC)?
Sunitinib
Targets VEGF and PDGF receptors.

Q69. Anticancer antibiotic not causing bone marrow suppression?
Bleomycin
Unique among cytotoxics.

Q70. Prophylaxis against TLS (tumor lysis syndrome)?
Allopurinol + hydration
Prevents uric acid nephropathy.

Q71. Drug used in pediatric ALL maintenance phase?
6-mercaptopurine
Along with methotrexate.

Q72. AML with t(15;17) treated with?
All-trans retinoic acid (ATRA)
Induces differentiation.

Q73. ATRA side effect?
Retinoic acid syndrome (fever, pulmonary infiltrates)
Requires steroids.

Q74. Oral alkylating agent used in gliomas?
Temozolomide
Crosses BBB.

Q75. Common TKI for GIST (c-kit positive tumors)?
Imatinib
Targets c-Kit and PDGFR.

Q76. DNA methyltransferase inhibitor used in MDS?
Azacitidine
Hypomethylates tumor suppressor genes.

Q77. EGFR TKI used in NSCLC with exon 19 deletion?
Erlotinib or gefitinib
Targeted oral therapy.

Q78. NSCLC with ALK rearrangement treated with?
Crizotinib
TKI targeting ALK.

Q79. TKI with adverse effect of visual disturbance (flashes)?
Crizotinib
Also hepatotoxicity.

Q80. Drug used in Hodgkin lymphoma and CD30+ tumors?
Brentuximab vedotin
Anti-CD30 antibody-drug conjugate.

Q81. Ipilimumab mechanism?
CTLA-4 inhibitor
Checkpoint inhibitor → immune activation.

Q82. PD-1 inhibitor examples?
Nivolumab, pembrolizumab
Used in melanoma, NSCLC, etc.

Q83. Major immune-related adverse effects of checkpoint inhibitors?
Pneumonitis, colitis, hepatitis
Due to autoimmune activation.

Q84. Use of dexrazoxane in chemotherapy?
Prevent doxorubicin cardiotoxicity
Iron chelator.

Q85. Common immunotherapy for prostate cancer (cell-based vaccine)?
Sipuleucel-T
Autologous dendritic cell vaccine.

Q86. Antifolate drug more potent than methotrexate?
Pemetrexed
Used in mesothelioma, NSCLC.

Q87. VEGF-A inhibitor causing proteinuria?
Bevacizumab
Monitor renal function.

Q88. Drug with specific toxicity: interstitial lung disease?
Bleomycin
Irreversible if not detected early.

Q89. Major resistance mechanism to methotrexate?
DHFR gene amplification
Leads to treatment failure.

Q90. Drug with S-phase specific arrest and cerebellar toxicity?
Cytarabine
High-dose monitoring required.

Q91. Chemo causing irreversible ototoxicity in children?
Cisplatin
Monitor hearing in pediatric cases.

Q92. Enzyme involved in activation of 5-FU?
Thymidine phosphorylase
Converts to active FdUMP.

Q93. Common side effect of etoposide?
Alopecia and myelosuppression
DNA strand breakage mechanism.

Q94. Newer TKI used in CML resistant to imatinib?
Dasatinib or nilotinib
Active in BCR-ABL mutations.

Q95. Platinum used in colorectal cancer regimens?
Oxaliplatin
Part of FOLFOX regimen.

Q96. Pegylated liposomal doxorubicin is used to?
Reduce cardiotoxicity
Alters pharmacokinetics.

Q97. Drug class of lenalidomide?
Immunomodulatory (IMiD) agent
Used in multiple myeloma, MDS.

Q98. Lenalidomide black box warning?
Teratogenicity
Structurally related to thalidomide.

Q99. Drug used in chemo-induced neutropenia recovery?
Filgrastim
Recombinant G-CSF.

Q100. Erythropoietin is contraindicated in which cancer?
Head and neck cancers receiving curative treatment
↑ Tumor progression risk.

Q101. Alkylating agent used in bone marrow ablation pre-transplant?
Busulfan
Causes profound myelosuppression.

Q102. 6-thioguanine is inactivated by?
Xanthine oxidase
Like 6-MP; caution with allopurinol.

Q103. 6-TG vs 6-MP: which is less affected by allopurinol?
6-thioguanine
Less dependent on xanthine oxidase.

Q104. Chemotherapy agent safe in renal failure?
Vincristine
Mainly hepatically cleared.

Q105. Hand-foot syndrome is most common with which drug?
Capecitabine
Redness, peeling, pain of palms/soles.

Q106. Most radiosensitizing anticancer drug?
5-Fluorouracil (5-FU)
Enhances radiation-induced DNA damage.

Q107. Prostate cancer drug with bone-protective effect?
Denosumab
RANKL inhibitor; prevents fractures.

Q108. Monoclonal antibody with progressive multifocal leukoencephalopathy (PML) risk?
Rituximab
Reactivation of JC virus.

Q109. Irinotecan major toxicity?
Severe diarrhea
Requires aggressive hydration and anticholinergics.

Q110. Metabolite of irinotecan causing toxicity?
SN-38
Potent active metabolite.

Q111. Enzyme deficiency increasing irinotecan toxicity?
UGT1A1
Reduced SN-38 clearance.

Q112. Topoisomerase I inhibitor used in colon cancer?
Irinotecan
FOLFIRI regimen.

Q113. Bortezomib mechanism of action?
Proteasome inhibition
Induces apoptosis in plasma cells.

Q114. Drug causing tumor flare reaction in prostate cancer?
Leuprolide (initially)
Add antiandrogen like flutamide initially.

Q115. Aromatase inhibitors not effective in?
Premenopausal women (monotherapy)
Require ovarian suppression.

Q116. Anticancer antibiotic most cardiotoxic?
Doxorubicin
Dose-dependent.

Q117. Alkylating agent useful in Hodgkin's lymphoma (ABVD regimen)?
Dacarbazine
Also part of MOPP.

Q118. Pro-drug requiring activation in liver for cytotoxicity?
Cyclophosphamide
Activated by CYP enzymes.

Q119. Chemo agent commonly causing hemorrhagic enteritis?
Melphalan
High-dose regimens.

Q120. Drug class causing alopecia, mucositis, myelosuppression?
Most antimetabolites
Especially 5-FU, methotrexate.

Q121. Drug used for high-dose methotrexate rescue?
Leucovorin
Folinic acid bypasses DHFR blockade.

Q122. Anticancer drug causing fatal hepatotoxicity with NSAIDs?
Methotrexate
Avoid combination.

Q123. Anticancer agent causing SIADH-like syndrome?
Vincristine
Also causes constipation and neuropathy.

Q124. GIST drug if imatinib-resistant?
Sunitinib
Also targets PDGF, VEGF.

Q125. Drug used for hepatocellular carcinoma (HCC)?
Sorafenib
Multi-kinase inhibitor.

Q126. Classic TKI causing skin rash as marker of efficacy?
Erlotinib
Acneiform rash correlates with response.

Q127. Anticancer drug contraindicated in pregnancy (most teratogenic)?
Methotrexate
Category X drug.

Q128. Drug used for hormone-refractory prostate cancer?
Enzalutamide
Androgen receptor antagonist.

Q129. Selective estrogen receptor degrader (SERD)?
Fulvestrant
Pure antagonist.

Q130. Monoclonal antibody with black box warning for bowel perforation?
Bevacizumab
Also poor wound healing.

Q131. Drug that prevents chemotherapy-induced nausea via NK1 receptor blockade?

Aprepitant
Blocks substance P pathway.

Q132. Drug class of olaparib?

PARP inhibitor
Used in BRCA-mutated cancers.

Q133. PARP inhibitors are synthetic lethal in?

BRCA-deficient cells
Accumulate DNA damage.

Q134. Drug used in relapsed/refractory multiple myeloma?

Carfilzomib
Second-gen proteasome inhibitor.

Q135. Key side effect of thalidomide/lenalidomide?

Thromboembolism
Prophylactic anticoagulation often needed.

Q136. Key toxicity of arsenic trioxide (APL therapy)?

QT prolongation
Monitor ECG.

Q137. Differentiation syndrome triggered by?

ATRA or arsenic trioxide
Steroids used for prevention.

Q138. Cytokine-release syndrome is associated with?

CAR-T cell therapy
Treat with tocilizumab (IL-6 blocker).

Q139. Anticancer monoclonal antibody for relapsed ALL (CD19+)?

Blinatumomab
BiTE antibody engaging T-cells.

Q140. MAB used for triple-negative breast cancer (PD-L1+)?

Atezolizumab
Combined with nab-paclitaxel.

Q141. ALK inhibitor used after crizotinib resistance?
Alectinib
Superior CNS penetration.

Q142. Major use of PEGylation in drug formulation?
Prolong half-life, reduce immunogenicity
Eg: PEG-asparaginase.

Q143. Asparaginase is used in?
ALL
Starves leukemic cells of asparagine.

Q144. Toxicity of asparaginase?
Pancreatitis, coagulopathy
Monitor amylase/lipase.

Q145. High-dose methotrexate monitoring requires?
Urine pH and serum levels
Alkalinization to avoid renal toxicity.

Q146. Drug causing hemorrhagic pericarditis and conjunctivitis?
Cytarabine (HiDAC)
Ocular toxicity with high doses.

Q147. Intrathecal drug causing paralysis if given IV accidentally?
Vincristine
Always label "For IV use only."

Q148. Anthracycline-induced heart failure is due to?
Free radical formation
Cumulative dose-related.

Q149. Drug causing red urine that is not hematuria?
Doxorubicin
Due to drug color, harmless.

Q150. DPD (dihydropyrimidine dehydrogenase) deficiency increases toxicity of?
5-FU
Screen in severe toxicity cases.

Q151. Key marker monitored in CML treatment response?
BCR-ABL transcript levels
Done via PCR.

Q152. TKI used in Philadelphia chromosome–positive ALL?
Dasatinib
Active in both CML and Ph+ ALL.

Q153. Common chemotherapeutic agent causing neurotoxicity + constipation?
Vincristine
Also causes SIADH.

Q154. Phase of cell cycle targeted by methotrexate?
S-phase
Antimetabolite.

Q155. Paclitaxel causes arrest in which phase?
M-phase
Inhibits microtubule depolymerization.

Q156. Drug that increases fetal hemoglobin in sickle cell disease?
Hydroxyurea
Also used in myeloproliferative disorders.

Q157. Antimetabolite causing cerebellar ataxia?
Cytarabine
High doses in AML.

Q158. Antimetabolite used in basal cell carcinoma (topical)?
5-FU cream
Applied locally.

Q159. Platinum agent causing severe nausea and vomiting?
Cisplatin
High emetogenic potential.

Q160. Oral SERM with agonist effect in bone?
Raloxifene
Used for osteoporosis and breast cancer prevention.

Q161. Recombinant uricase enzyme used in tumor lysis?
Rasburicase
Converts uric acid to allantoin.

Q162. Flu-like symptoms are common with which biologic?
Interferon-α
Used in melanoma, CML, renal cell carcinoma.

Q163. Target of trastuzumab?
HER2/neu
Tyrosine kinase receptor.

Q164. HER2+ breast cancer, brain metastasis – preferred treatment?
Lapatinib
TKI with CNS penetration.

Q165. Docetaxel vs paclitaxel – which has more fluid retention?
Docetaxel
Premedicate with steroids.

Q166. Oral TKI used in thyroid cancer (RET mutation)?
Vandetanib
QT prolongation risk.

Q167. Antibody–drug conjugate used in HER2+ breast cancer?
T-DM1 (trastuzumab emtansine)
Antibody + cytotoxic agent.

Q168. Which kinase does sorafenib inhibit?
RAF kinase + VEGFR
Used in HCC, RCC.

Q169. Cell cycle–nonspecific agent among antineoplastics?
Alkylating agents
Eg: cyclophosphamide.

Q170. Folate antagonist safe in choriocarcinoma?
Methotrexate
Also used in ectopic pregnancy.

Q171. Drug class most associated with cumulative dose–dependent cardiotoxicity?
Anthracyclines
Doxorubicin, daunorubicin.

Q172. Main elimination route of methotrexate?
Renal
Avoid in renal failure.

Q173. Target of pembrolizumab?
PD-1 receptor
Boosts T-cell activity.

Q174. Drug that may cause autoimmune endocrinopathy (thyroiditis, adrenalitis)?
Immune checkpoint inhibitors
Eg: nivolumab, pembrolizumab.

Q175. Agent most likely to cause hemorrhagic colitis?
Bevacizumab
Bowel perforation also possible.

Q176. Anticancer agent associated with posterior reversible encephalopathy syndrome (PRES)?
Cyclosporine, tacrolimus, bevacizumab
Visual symptoms + seizures.

Q177. Agent used in hormone-sensitive endometrial carcinoma?
Megestrol acetate
Progestin therapy.

Q178. Epothilone analog used in taxane-resistant cancers?
Ixabepilone
M-phase active.

Q179. Oral fluoropyrimidine commonly used in GI cancers?
Capecitabine
Prodrug of 5-FU.

Q180. Chemo drug with highest emetogenic potential?
Cisplatin
Requires triple antiemetic prophylaxis.

Q181. Cytotoxic drug causing hemorrhagic pericarditis?
Cyclophosphamide
Rare, dose-related.

Q182. Enzyme that activates cyclophosphamide?
CYP2B6
Hepatic activation.

Q183. Agent used to mobilize stem cells before autologous transplant?
G-CSF (filgrastim)
Enhances peripheral CD34+ cells.

Q184. CD52-targeted monoclonal antibody in CLL?
Alemtuzumab
Profound immunosuppression.

Q185. Oral prodrug of cytarabine?
None
Cytarabine is IV only; oral absorption poor.

Q186. Inhibitor of hedgehog signaling in basal cell carcinoma?
Vismodegib
Used in advanced BCC.

Q187. Tyrosine kinase mutation resistant to imatinib?
T315I
Responds to ponatinib.

Q188. Oral arsenic derivative used in APL?
Arsenic trioxide
Combined with ATRA.

Q189. Drug combination with high TLS risk?
R-CHOP (for large B-cell lymphoma)
Requires monitoring and prophylaxis.

Q190. Antimetabolite causing pigmentation of palms and mucosa?
5-FU
Also hand-foot syndrome.

Q191. S-phase specific agent causing conjunctivitis?
Cytarabine
Prophylactic eye drops needed.

Q192. Drug class for triple-negative breast cancer (BRCA+)?
PARP inhibitors
Olaparib, talazoparib.

Q193. Topoisomerase II inhibitors increase risk of?
Secondary AML
Especially etoposide, doxorubicin.

Q194. Drug used for methotrexate overdose?
Glucarpidase
Enzyme that breaks down MTX.

Q195. VEGF inhibitor contraindicated post-surgery?
Bevacizumab
Delay at least 28 days post-op.

Q196. Drug inhibiting CDK4/6 in breast cancer?
Palbociclib
Arrests cells at G1-S phase.

Q197. Oral proteasome inhibitor in multiple myeloma?
Ixazomib
Weekly dosing regimen.

Q198. Most potent agent against CNS leukemia (ALL)?
Methotrexate (intrathecal)
Prophylaxis and treatment.

Q199. Pegylated asparaginase benefits?
Longer half-life, fewer allergic reactions
Preferred in many protocols.

Q200. Key risk when combining anthracyclines with trastuzumab?
Synergistic cardiotoxicity
Monitor LVEF closely.

Respiratory Pharmacology

Q1. Drug of choice for acute severe asthma?
Salbutamol (short-acting β2-agonist)
Rapid bronchodilation.

Q2. Long-acting β2-agonist used for maintenance therapy in asthma?
Salmeterol
Not for acute relief.

Q3. Anticholinergic bronchodilator used in COPD?
Tiotropium
Long-acting muscarinic antagonist.

Q4. Short-acting anticholinergic agent used in acute asthma exacerbation?
Ipratropium bromide
Often combined with salbutamol.

Q5. Inhaled corticosteroid commonly used in asthma maintenance?
Budesonide or fluticasone
Reduces airway inflammation.

Q6. Major side effect of inhaled corticosteroids?
Oral candidiasis
Use spacer and rinse mouth.

Q7. Leukotriene receptor antagonist used in asthma?
Montelukast
Effective in aspirin-sensitive asthma.

Q8. 5-lipoxygenase inhibitor in asthma?
Zileuton
Blocks leukotriene synthesis.

Q9. Monoclonal antibody against IgE?
Omalizumab
Used in severe allergic asthma.

Q10. Drug that relaxes bronchial smooth muscle via PDE inhibition?
Theophylline
Narrow therapeutic index.

Q11. Theophylline toxicity symptoms?
Nausea, tremors, seizures
Monitor serum levels.

Q12. Mucolytic agent used in COPD?
N-acetylcysteine
Breaks disulfide bonds in mucus.

Q13. Expectorant commonly used in cough?
Guaifenesin
Increases respiratory tract secretions.

Q14. Antitussive acting on medullary cough center?
Dextromethorphan
Non-opioid cough suppressant.

Q15. Opioid used in dry, non-productive cough?
Codeine
Centrally suppresses cough reflex.

Q16. Drug class contraindicated in acute asthma?
β-blockers
May cause bronchospasm.

Q17. Drug used for prevention of exercise-induced bronchospasm?
Salbutamol (pre-exercise)
Or leukotriene antagonists.

Q18. Most effective treatment for COPD exacerbation?
Short-acting bronchodilators + corticosteroids
Often with antibiotics.

Q19. Preferred oxygen therapy target SpO_2 in COPD?
88–92%
To prevent CO2 retention.

Q20. First-line therapy for stable COPD with frequent symptoms?
LABA + LAMA combination
Long-acting agents preferred.

Q21. Inhaled corticosteroids in COPD are used for?
Frequent exacerbations
Not as monotherapy.

Q22. Phosphodiesterase-4 inhibitor used in COPD?
Roflumilast
Reduces exacerbations.

Q23. Side effect of roflumilast?
Weight loss, GI symptoms
Monitor in elderly.

Q24. MAB targeting IL-5 in eosinophilic asthma?
Mepolizumab
Reduces eosinophilic inflammation.

Q25. Inhaler technique device to improve corticosteroid delivery?
Spacer
Reduces oropharyngeal deposition.

Q26. Step-up therapy in uncontrolled asthma includes?
Increase ICS dose or add LABA
Follow GINA guidelines.

Q27. Drug causing paradoxical bronchospasm?
Inhaled β-agonists (rare)
Stop use if occurs.

Q28. Drug safe in asthma during pregnancy?
Inhaled budesonide
Category B.

Q29. Drug of choice for nocturnal asthma?
Sustained-release theophylline or salmeterol
Long-acting bronchodilators.

Q30. Monoclonal antibody blocking IL-4/IL-13 pathway?
Dupilumab
Used in moderate-to-severe asthma.

Q31. Monoclonal antibody targeting IL-13 in asthma?
Lebrikizumab
Used in allergic asthma.

Q32. Antihistamine useful in allergic rhinitis with asthma?
Cetirizine or loratadine
Reduces allergic triggers.

Q33. Nasal corticosteroid used in allergic rhinitis?
Fluticasone nasal spray
Anti-inflammatory action.

Q34. First-line treatment for mild intermittent asthma?
Low-dose ICS as needed or SABA
Per GINA guidelines.

Q35. Leukotriene receptor antagonist with once-daily dosing?
Montelukast
Oral administration.

Q36. Theophylline interacts with which drugs?
Erythromycin, ciprofloxacin, phenytoin
Alters metabolism.

Q37. Antiasthmatic drug with narrow therapeutic index?
Theophylline
Monitor plasma levels.

Q38. Most effective single controller for persistent asthma?
Inhaled corticosteroids
Reduce airway hyperreactivity.

Q39. Preferred route for bronchodilator in acute asthma?
Inhalation
Direct and faster effect.

Q40. Preferred corticosteroid for oral burst therapy in asthma?
Prednisolone
Short course for exacerbation.

Q41. Asthma severity classification is based on?
Frequency of symptoms and PEF values
Used for treatment steps.

Q42. LABA alone in asthma increases risk of?
Asthma-related deaths
Always combine with ICS.

Q43. Preferred treatment in COPD with eosinophilia?
ICS + LABA
Inflammation-guided therapy.

Q44. Inhaled corticosteroids may increase risk of?
Pneumonia (in COPD)
Use only if indicated.

Q45. Asthma vs COPD reversibility test?
Spirometry after bronchodilator
Asthma is reversible.

Q46. Best bronchodilator for exercise-induced bronchospasm?
Salbutamol (before exercise)
Prevents bronchospasm.

Q47. Most common trigger for asthma exacerbation?
Respiratory viral infections
Rhinovirus common.

Q48. Antiasthmatic monoclonal antibody given subcutaneously every 2–4 weeks?
Omalizumab
For severe IgE-mediated asthma.

Q49. Marker used to assess eosinophilic airway inflammation?
FeNO (Fractional exhaled nitric oxide)
Non-invasive.

Q50. Role of peak flow meter in asthma?
Monitoring PEF variability
Self-monitoring tool.

Q50. Biologic used in severe allergic asthma (IgE mediated)?
Omalizumab
Anti-IgE monoclonal antibody.

Q51. Omalizumab route of administration?
Subcutaneous injection
Given every 2–4 weeks.

Q52. Biologic used in eosinophilic asthma?
Mepolizumab
Anti–IL-5 monoclonal antibody.

Q53. Antitussive with central action?
Dextromethorphan
NMDA receptor antagonist, non-opioid.

Q54. Codeine is avoided in children because?
Risk of respiratory depression
Especially ultra-rapid CYP2D6 metabolizers.

Q55. Peripheral antitussive with demulcent action?
Honey or glycerin-based lozenges
Soothe mucosa and reduce cough reflex.

Q56. Expectorant that stimulates bronchial secretion?
Guaifenesin
Helps in productive cough by thinning mucus.

Q57. Drug of choice for allergic rhinitis?
Intranasal corticosteroids
Eg: mometasone, fluticasone.

Q58. First-generation antihistamine used in allergic rhinitis?
Chlorpheniramine
Causes sedation, short-acting.

Q59. Second-generation antihistamines used for rhinitis?
Loratadine, cetirizine
Longer acting, non-sedating.

Q60. Nasal decongestant that causes rebound congestion?
Oxymetazoline
Prolonged use leads to rhinitis medicamentosa.

Q61. Long-term use of nasal decongestants can cause?
Tachyphylaxis and rebound nasal congestion
Limit use to ≤5 days.

Q62. Cromolyn sodium mechanism?
Mast cell stabilizer
Prevents degranulation, used in allergic asthma.

Q63. Cromolyn sodium limitation?
Not effective for acute asthma
Used prophylactically only.

Q64. Antihistamine with least sedation?
Fexofenadine
Poor CNS penetration.

Q65. Drug used in cystic fibrosis to clear mucus?
Dornase alfa (DNase enzyme)
Breaks down DNA in thick mucus.

Q66. Drug enhancing CFTR function in cystic fibrosis?
Ivacaftor
Improves chloride channel gating.

Q67. Macrolide used chronically in cystic fibrosis?
Azithromycin
Anti-inflammatory and antimicrobial effect.

Q68. Main antimicrobial used in Pseudomonas colonization (CF)?
Inhaled tobramycin
Aminoglycoside antibiotic.

Q69. Antitubercular drug causing orange discoloration of secretions?
Rifampin
No clinical concern, but counseling needed.

Q70. Antitubercular drug causing optic neuritis?
Ethambutol
Monitor visual acuity, especially color vision.

Q71. DOC for latent TB infection?
Isoniazid for 6–9 months
Alternative: rifampin x 4 months.

Q72. Antitubercular drug needing B6 supplementation?
Isoniazid
Prevents peripheral neuropathy.

Q73. Pyrazinamide side effect?
Hyperuricemia
May precipitate gout.

Q74. First-line regimen for pulmonary TB (initial 2 months)?
HRZE: Isoniazid, Rifampin, Pyrazinamide, Ethambutol
Followed by HR for 4 months.

Q75. Fixed-dose combinations are used in TB to?
Improve compliance and reduce resistance
Less chance of selective monotherapy.

Q76. Second-line injectable drug in MDR-TB?
Amikacin or kanamycin
Ototoxicity and nephrotoxicity are concerns.

Q77. Fluoroquinolone used in MDR-TB?
Levofloxacin or moxifloxacin
Active against Mycobacterium tuberculosis.

Q78. Drug used for extensively drug-resistant TB (XDR-TB)?
Bedaquiline
Inhibits mycobacterial ATP synthase.

Q79. Bedaquiline side effect?
QT prolongation
Requires ECG monitoring.

Q80. Delamanid in TB acts by?
Inhibiting mycolic acid synthesis
Used in MDR-TB treatment.

Q81. ADRs common to both isoniazid and rifampin?
Hepatotoxicity
Monitor liver enzymes during therapy.

Q82. TB drug associated with lupus-like syndrome?
Isoniazid
Rare but exam-favorite ADR.

Q83. TB drug used in pregnancy with caution?
Isoniazid (with pyridoxine)
Safe if monitored.

Q84. Rifampin induces which enzyme system?
CYP450
Reduces effectiveness of oral contraceptives, warfarin.

Q85. Prophylaxis after contact with TB patient (child <5 yrs)?
Isoniazid for 6 months
Even without active disease signs.

Q86. Anti-TB drug with bactericidal action in acidic pH (inside macrophages)?

Pyrazinamide

Effective in latent bacilli.

Q87. Antitubercular drug requiring eye exams?

Ethambutol

Dose-related optic toxicity.

Q88. Drug interactions of rifampin?

↓ Effect of many drugs (OC pills, warfarin, ART)

Due to CYP induction.

Q89. Rifabutin vs rifampin in HIV patients?

Rifabutin preferred

Less CYP induction = better ART compatibility.

Q90. Ethionamide is a second-line TB drug similar to?

Isoniazid

Same target (InhA) but more side effects.

Q91. Anti-TB drug with the most potent sterilizing effect on semi-dormant bacilli?

Rifampin

Kills slowly replicating intracellular organisms.

Q92. Fixed-dose combination for TB is used to prevent?

Monotherapy and resistance

Also improves compliance.

Q93. Most common cause of TB treatment failure?

Poor compliance

Leads to drug resistance.

Q94. Which drug inhibits ATP synthase in mycobacteria?

Bedaquiline

Used in MDR-TB.

Q95. Drug used in TB meningitis with good CNS penetration?

Isoniazid

Along with pyrazinamide and rifampin.

Q96. Which antitubercular drug causes gout-like symptoms?
Pyrazinamide
Due to hyperuricemia.

Q97. Drug causing reddish-orange discoloration of tears, urine, sweat?
Rifampin
Harmless but alarming to patients.

Q98. Which TB drug causes hypersensitivity and interstitial nephritis?
Streptomycin
Also causes ototoxicity.

Q99. Which fluoroquinolone is most active against TB?
Moxifloxacin
Used in drug-resistant TB.

Q100. Mechanism of action of isoniazid?
Inhibits mycolic acid synthesis
Bactericidal for actively dividing bacilli.

Q101. Mutation in KatG gene causes resistance to?
Isoniazid
KatG activates INH.

Q102. Drug causing red-green color blindness?
Ethambutol
Optic neuritis.

Q103. Anti-TB drug not used in children due to visual toxicity?
Ethambutol
Not recommended <5 years old.

Q104. First-line TB drug most associated with hepatotoxicity?
Pyrazinamide
Monitor LFTs regularly.

Q105. Drug that enhances the toxicity of isoniazid?
Rifampin
Additive hepatotoxicity.

Q106. Antitubercular drug not safe in pregnancy (unless essential)?
Streptomycin
Ototoxic to fetus.

Q107. Drug with both bactericidal and sterilizing action in TB?
Rifampin
Also active in latent TB.

Q108. Mechanism of ethambutol?
Inhibits arabinosyl transferase
Affects cell wall polymerization.

Q109. Primary reason for using pyrazinamide only in intensive phase?
Maximal activity in acidic pH
Helps early sterilization.

Q110. Risk factor for INH-induced peripheral neuropathy?
Diabetes, alcohol, malnutrition
Supplement with pyridoxine.

Q111. DOC for non-tuberculous Mycobacterium avium complex (MAC)?
Azithromycin + ethambutol
With or without rifabutin.

Q112. Preferred TB regimen in HIV patients?
HRZE with cotrimoxazole prophylaxis
Rifabutin preferred over rifampin if on ART.

Q113. Rifampin drug interaction with antiretrovirals is due to?
CYP3A4 induction
Lowers ART levels.

Q114. Adverse effect of delamanid?
QT prolongation
Like bedaquiline.

Q115. BCG vaccine contains?
Live attenuated Mycobacterium bovis
Prevents severe forms of childhood TB.

Q116. BCG is contraindicated in?
Immunodeficient children
Risk of disseminated infection.

Q117. Which anti-TB drug inhibits RNA synthesis?
Rifampin
Binds β-subunit of RNA polymerase.

Q118. Bedaquiline used for which type of TB?
MDR-TB and XDR-TB
In combination regimens.

Q119. Mechanism of action of delamanid?
Inhibits mycolic acid synthesis
Used in resistant TB.

Q120. Major advantage of daily DOTS therapy?
Improves adherence
Reduces emergence of resistance.

Q121. Most important goal of asthma therapy?
Prevent exacerbations and maintain normal activity
Along with minimal use of rescue meds.

Q122. Step-up therapy in asthma is based on?
Frequency and severity of symptoms
Guided by GINA guidelines.

Q123. Step-down asthma therapy is considered when?
Symptoms controlled for 3 months
Reduce steroid burden.

Q124. SMART therapy in asthma stands for?
Single Maintenance And Reliever Therapy
ICS + formoterol used for both.

Q125. Preferred reliever in GINA guidelines for moderate asthma?
Low-dose ICS-formoterol
Safer than SABA alone.

Q126. Oral corticosteroid used in severe acute asthma?
Prednisolone
Short course (5–7 days) as burst therapy.

Q127. Methylprednisolone vs dexamethasone: which has longer half-life?
Dexamethasone
Used in 1–2 dose regimens for asthma.

Q128. Biologic for severe asthma with elevated eosinophils?
Benralizumab
IL-5 receptor antagonist.

Q129. Antileukotriene drug used for allergic rhinitis + asthma?
Montelukast
Once-daily oral dose.

Q130. Leukotriene involved in bronchoconstriction and mucus secretion?
LTD4
Blocked by montelukast.

Q131. Inhaler device preferred in children <5 years?
Metered-dose inhaler with spacer
Ensures effective delivery.

Q132. Nebulized β2 agonist of choice for acute asthma?
Salbutamol
Quick onset.

Q133. Drug class of roflumilast?
PDE-4 inhibitor
Used in severe COPD.

Q134. Roflumilast side effects?
Weight loss, diarrhea
GI upset common.

Q135. Role of macrolides in COPD?
Anti-inflammatory, reduce exacerbations
Azithromycin in chronic use.

Q136. Drug contraindicated in asthma due to bronchospasm risk?
NSAIDs (especially aspirin)
AERD (aspirin-exacerbated respiratory disease).

Q137. Drug class of ephedrine?
Mixed-acting sympathomimetic
Causes vasoconstriction and bronchodilation.

Q138. Preferred antihistamine in pregnancy?
Loratadine
Non-sedating, category B.

Q139. Common preservative in nebulizer solution causing bronchospasm?
Benzalkonium chloride
Rare but possible reaction.

Q140. Oxygen therapy is indicated when PaO_2 < ?

<55 mmHg (or SaO_2 $<88\%$)

Long-term oxygen improves survival in COPD.

Q141. Oxygen therapy target in COPD?

88–92% saturation

Avoid hyperoxia and CO_2 retention.

Q142. Domiciliary oxygen therapy duration for benefit?

>15 hours/day

Reduces pulmonary hypertension.

Q143. Mucolytic with antioxidant properties?

N-acetylcysteine (NAC)

Also used as hepatoprotective.

Q144. Nonselective PDE inhibitor used as bronchodilator?

Theophylline

Narrow therapeutic window.

Q145. Theophylline toxicity includes?

Seizures, arrhythmias, GI upset

Requires serum monitoring.

Q146. Drugs increasing theophylline levels?

Erythromycin, ciprofloxacin

Inhibit metabolism.

Q147. Drugs decreasing theophylline levels?

Phenytoin, phenobarbital, smoking

Induce metabolism.

Q148. Anticholinergic that blocks M3 receptor in airways?

Tiotropium

Long-acting bronchodilator in COPD.

Q149. ICS preferred in pediatric asthma for safety?

Budesonide

Least growth suppression.

Q150. COPD classification includes which major parameters?

FEV_1, symptoms, exacerbation history

GOLD guidelines.

Q151. Drug used to prevent altitude sickness?
Acetazolamide
Carbonic anhydrase inhibitor → mild acidosis → stimulates respiration.

Q152. Mechanism of acetazolamide in altitude sickness?
Induces metabolic acidosis
Stimulates central respiratory drive.

Q153. Drug used for high altitude pulmonary edema (HAPE)?
Nifedipine
Reduces pulmonary artery pressure.

Q154. PDE-5 inhibitor used in pulmonary arterial hypertension (PAH)?
Sildenafil
Causes pulmonary vasodilation.

Q155. Endothelin receptor antagonist used in PAH?
Bosentan
Blocks ET-A and ET-B receptors.

Q156. Major adverse effect of bosentan?
Hepatotoxicity
Monitor liver enzymes monthly.

Q157. Prostacyclin analog used in PAH?
Epoprostenol
Administered via continuous IV infusion.

Q158. Main limitation of epoprostenol?
Short half-life, requires continuous infusion
Risk of rebound pulmonary hypertension on interruption.

Q159. Inhaled prostacyclin analog in PAH?
Iloprost
Used 6–9 times daily.

Q160. Oral prostacyclin receptor agonist for PAH?
Selexipag
Better compliance than iloprost.

Q161. Target of riociguat in PAH?
Stimulates soluble guanylate cyclase
Enhances NO pathway.

Q162. Drug contraindicated with nitrates due to risk of hypotension?
Sildenafil
Both increase cGMP → severe hypotension.

Q163. Role of nitric oxide inhalation in neonatal care?
Pulmonary vasodilation in persistent pulmonary hypertension of newborn
Selective pulmonary effect.

Q164. Long-acting inhaled β2 agonist used once daily in COPD?
Indacaterol
Ultra-long-acting bronchodilator.

Q165. Combination inhaler in COPD with LABA + LAMA?
Formoterol + tiotropium or indacaterol + glycopyrronium
Dual bronchodilation.

Q166. Triple therapy inhaler in COPD contains?
LABA + LAMA + ICS
Improves symptoms and reduces exacerbations.

Q167. Cough suppressant contraindicated in productive cough?
Dextromethorphan
May lead to mucus retention.

Q168. Mast cell stabilizer used in exercise-induced asthma?
Cromolyn sodium
Preventive, not for acute use.

Q169. Key difference between asthma and COPD response to steroids?
Asthma: good response; COPD: limited response
Due to different inflammatory profiles.

Q170. COPD patients most likely to benefit from ICS if?
Eosinophil count is high (>300 cells/μL)
Predicts steroid responsiveness.

Q171. Smoking induces which enzyme affecting drug metabolism?
CYP1A2
Reduces efficacy of theophylline.

Q172. Drug-induced interstitial lung disease is seen with?
Amiodarone, methotrexate, bleomycin
Monitor pulmonary symptoms.

Q173. Drug causing nasal mucosal atrophy with long-term use?
Nasal decongestants (e.g., oxymetazoline)
Due to vasoconstriction.

Q174. Drug causing paroxysmal dry cough in 10–20% patients?
ACE inhibitors (e.g., enalapril)
Due to bradykinin accumulation.

Q175. Preferred alternative to ACE inhibitors in cough-prone patients?
ARBs (e.g., losartan)
No bradykinin effect.

Q176. Inhaler device preferred in elderly with poor coordination?
Dry powder inhaler (DPI) or nebulizer
Easier technique.

Q177. Main non-pharmacological therapy in COPD?
Smoking cessation
Slows disease progression.

Q178. Drug used in cystic fibrosis to hydrate airway mucus?
Hypertonic saline inhalation
Increases airway surface liquid.

Q179. Preferred therapy for severe asthma not controlled on ICS + LABA?
Add biologic (e.g., omalizumab or mepolizumab)
Based on phenotype.

Q180. Which drug class is contraindicated in aspirin-exacerbated respiratory disease (AERD)?
NSAIDs (esp. aspirin)
Leukotriene inhibitors preferred.

Q181. Which drug is used to reduce ventilator-associated pneumonia risk in ICU patients?
Chlorhexidine oral care
Reduces oropharyngeal colonization.

Q182. Drug used for cough suppression in pulmonary tuberculosis?
Codeine
Helps symptomatic relief (with caution).

Q183. Long-term use of ICS in children may affect?
Linear growth
Monitor height annually.

Q184. Key ADR of mepolizumab (anti–IL-5)?
Hypersensitivity reactions
Includes urticaria and angioedema.

Q185. Which inhaler component improves deposition in lungs?
Spacer
Reduces oropharyngeal deposition.

Q186. Beta-agonist overuse in asthma may lead to?
Tachyphylaxis and arrhythmia
Receptor downregulation.

Q187. Best parameter to monitor asthma control at home?
Peak expiratory flow rate (PEFR)
Daily tracking with peak flow meter.

Q188. Which mucolytic agent targets disulfide bonds in mucus?
N-acetylcysteine
Reduces mucus viscosity.

Q189. Which is a danger sign in a patient using SABAs frequently?
>2 uses/week
Indicates poor asthma control.

Q190. Salmeterol onset of action is?
Slow (20–30 minutes)
Not for acute relief.

Q191. Mechanism of ipratropium in COPD?
Blocks M3 receptors → bronchodilation
Reduces vagal tone.

Q192. Antileukotriene that causes Churg-Strauss syndrome rarely?
Montelukast
Monitor eosinophil count.

Q193. Preferred bronchodilator in acute bronchospasm?
Salbutamol (inhaled)
Rapid action via β2 stimulation.

Q194. Drug used as premedication before bronchial challenge test?
Anticholinergic or SABA
Reduces risk of severe response.

Q195. Role of ketotifen in respiratory disease?
Mast cell stabilizer in asthma prophylaxis
Rarely used today.

Q196. Drug that improves mucociliary clearance in bronchiectasis?
Hypertonic saline or dornase alfa
Loosens mucus plugs.

Q197. Main goal of asthma action plan?
Empower patient to self-manage exacerbations
Includes peak flow zones.

Q198. Best predictor of mortality in COPD?
FEV1
Lower value = higher risk.

Q199. Preferred first-line TB treatment for DOTS Category I?
2HRZE/4HR
2 months of intensive + 4 months continuation.

Q200. Which respiratory drug needs serum level monitoring?
Theophylline
Narrow therapeutic window.

Gastrointestinal Pharmacology

Q1. Drug class most effective for healing peptic ulcers?
Proton pump inhibitors (PPIs)
Eg: omeprazole, pantoprazole.

Q2. PPI mechanism of action?
Irreversible inhibition of H^+/K^+-ATPase
Final step of acid secretion.

Q3. Best time to administer PPIs?
30–60 minutes before meals
Maximal effect on active proton pumps.

Q4. Common adverse effect of long-term PPI use?
Hypomagnesemia, fractures, B12 deficiency
Due to reduced absorption.

Q5. H_2 blockers act by?
Blocking histamine (H2) receptors on parietal cells
Eg: ranitidine, famotidine.

Q6. H_2 blocker with antiandrogenic effects?
Cimetidine
Causes gynecomastia and impotence.

Q7. Drug that neutralizes acid in stomach directly?
Antacids
Eg: magnesium hydroxide, calcium carbonate.

Q8. Antacid causing constipation?
Aluminum hydroxide
Slows intestinal motility.

Q9. Antacid causing diarrhea?
Magnesium hydroxide
Stimulates GI motility.

Q10. Antacid interaction with tetracycline or fluoroquinolones?
Chelation reduces absorption
Separate dosing required.

Q11. Sucralfate mechanism?
Forms protective barrier over ulcers
Binds to exposed proteins.

Q12. Sucralfate should be avoided with?
PPIs or antacids
Needs acidic pH to work.

Q13. Misoprostol mechanism of action?
PGE1 analog – increases mucus, reduces acid
Used for NSAID-induced ulcers.

Q14. Major side effect of misoprostol?
Diarrhea
Also causes abdominal cramping.

Q15. Misoprostol contraindicated in?
Pregnancy
Causes uterine contractions → abortion.

Q16. Bismuth compounds are used in?
H. pylori eradication regimens
Also have antimicrobial effects.

Q17. Triple therapy for H. pylori includes?
PPI + amoxicillin + clarithromycin
For 14 days.

Q18. Quadruple therapy includes?
PPI + bismuth + metronidazole + tetracycline
Used when clarithromycin resistance is high.

Q19. Best regimen for refractory H. pylori infection?
Bismuth quadruple therapy
14-day course.

Q20. Drug class used to treat motion sickness?
Antihistamines (H1 blockers) and anticholinergics
Eg: meclizine, scopolamine.

Q21. Antiemetic for chemotherapy-induced vomiting?
Ondansetron
5-HT3 receptor antagonist.

Q22. Major side effect of ondansetron?
QT interval prolongation
Caution in cardiac patients.

Q23. Neurokinin-1 (NK1) antagonist used in vomiting?
Aprepitant
Blocks substance P pathway.

Q24. D2 receptor antagonist used for nausea and gastroparesis?
Metoclopramide
Increases GI motility.

Q25. Metoclopramide contraindicated in?
Parkinson's disease
Worsens extrapyramidal symptoms.

Q26. Domperidone vs metoclopramide?
Domperidone doesn't cross BBB
Fewer CNS side effects.

Q27. Laxative used in hepatic encephalopathy?
Lactulose
Acidifies colon, traps ammonia.

Q28. Osmotic purgative for bowel prep?
Polyethylene glycol (PEG)
Balanced electrolyte solution.

Q29. Bulk-forming laxatives example?
Psyllium
Increase stool bulk and water content.

Q30. Stool softener safe in pregnancy?
Docusate sodium
Mild, surfactant action.

Q31. Stimulant laxative that may cause dependence?
Bisacodyl
Increases intestinal motility.

Q32. Laxative that can cause melanosis coli?
Senna
Benign pigmentation of colon.

Q33. Drug used to treat opioid-induced constipation?
Methylnaltrexone
Peripheral μ-receptor antagonist.

Q34. Lubiprostone mechanism?
Activates chloride channels (CIC-2)
Increases intestinal fluid.

Q35. Linaclotide used for?
IBS-C (constipation predominant)
Guanylate cyclase-C agonist.

Q36. Loperamide is a?
Peripheral opioid agonist
Used as antidiarrheal.

Q37. Loperamide contraindicated in?
Infectious/bloody diarrhea
May worsen disease.

Q38. Bile acid sequestrant used in bile acid diarrhea?
Cholestyramine
Binds bile salts.

Q39. Antimotility agent contraindicated in children <2 years?
Diphenoxylate-atropine
Risk of respiratory depression.

Q40. Most effective drug for chemotherapy vomiting?
5-HT3 antagonist + NK1 antagonist + steroid
Triple regimen.

Q41. Corticosteroid used as antiemetic?
Dexamethasone
Used with 5-HT3 blockers.

Q42. Cannabinoid used in chemotherapy nausea?
Dronabinol
Appetite stimulation + antiemesis.

Q43. Antacid causing milk-alkali syndrome?
Calcium carbonate
Hypercalcemia + alkalosis.

Q44. Drug causing rebound acid hypersecretion on withdrawal?
PPIs
Tapering advised after prolonged use.

Q45. Treatment for Zollinger-Ellison syndrome?
High-dose PPIs
Eg: omeprazole, esomeprazole.

Q46. H2 blocker safe in pregnancy?
Ranitidine (historically), now: famotidine
Less teratogenic risk.

Q47. Laxative avoided in renal failure due to Mg overload?
Magnesium salts
Risk of hypermagnesemia.

Q48. Drug-induced pancreatitis is caused by?
Valproate, azathioprine, thiazides
Rare but serious.

Q49. Antibiotic used in hepatic encephalopathy?
Rifaximin
Reduces ammonia-producing gut flora.

Q50. Drug for irritable bowel syndrome with diarrhea (IBS-D)?
Alosetron
5-HT3 antagonist (restricted use due to ischemic colitis).

Q51. Which drug activates guanylate cyclase-C to treat chronic constipation?
Linaclotide
Increases chloride and water secretion in intestine.

Q52. Which drug is a μ-opioid receptor antagonist used for post-op ileus?
Alvimopan
Shortens GI recovery time.

Q53. Which antiemetic is effective in anticipatory nausea?
Lorazepam
Benzodiazepine—anxiolytic and amnestic effects.

Q54. Which laxative class increases stool water via osmotic action?
Osmotic laxatives
Eg: lactulose, magnesium salts, PEG.

Q55. Laxative that works fastest?
Rectal bisacodyl or phosphate enema
Acts within minutes to hours.

Q56. Drug used in IBS with constipation and bloating?
Linaclotide
Improves bowel movements and reduces pain.

Q57. MOA of lubiprostone in constipation?
Activates type-2 chloride channels (CIC-2)
Increases intestinal fluid.

Q58. Antidiarrheal safe in travelers' diarrhea (non-bloody)?
Loperamide
Only if no fever or blood in stool.

Q59. Main difference between metoclopramide and domperidone?
Domperidone has less CNS toxicity
Does not cross BBB effectively.

Q60. Drug used for portal systemic encephalopathy?
Lactulose
Reduces ammonia absorption in gut.

Q61. Drug that may precipitate ischemic colitis in IBS treatment?
Alosetron
Use restricted to women with severe IBS-D.

Q62. Laxative safe for long-term use in elderly?
Bulk-forming laxatives (e.g., psyllium)
Mimic dietary fiber.

Q63. Which antacid causes milk-alkali syndrome if overused with calcium?
Calcium carbonate
Results in hypercalcemia + alkalosis.

Q64. Chronic use of antacids may lead to?
Electrolyte imbalance
Alkalosis, hypophosphatemia, diarrhea or constipation.

Q65. Mucosal protective agent not absorbed systemically?
Sucralfate
Acts locally on ulcer base.

Q66. Drug contraindicated with PPI due to interaction?
Clopidogrel (especially with omeprazole)
Reduces clopidogrel activation via CYP2C19 inhibition.

Q67. Best diagnostic test to confirm H. pylori infection eradication?
Urea breath test
High sensitivity and specificity.

Q68. Antibiotic resistance in H. pylori is most common with?
Clarithromycin
Fails triple therapy.

Q69. First-line therapy for H. pylori in areas with high resistance?
Bismuth-based quadruple therapy
Alternative: sequential or concomitant therapy.

Q70. Drug combination for eradication of H. pylori?
PPI + 2 antibiotics (usually clarithromycin + amoxicillin)
Add bismuth or metronidazole in resistant cases.

Q71. 5-HT3 antagonist causing constipation as side effect?
Ondansetron
Especially with long-term use.

Q72. Dopamine antagonist with risk of extrapyramidal effects?
Metoclopramide
Dystonia, Parkinsonism, tardive dyskinesia.

Q73. GI prokinetic with least CNS side effects?
Itopride
Low CNS penetration.

Q74. Antacid contraindicated in renal failure?
Magnesium and aluminum salts
Risk of accumulation and toxicity.

Q75. Most effective agent to prevent NSAID-induced ulcer?
PPI
Superior to H2 blockers or misoprostol.

Q76. Drug that acts both as antacid and adsorbent in diarrhea?
Bismuth subsalicylate
Antimicrobial and anti-secretory effects.

Q77. Agent used in bile acid–induced diarrhea post-cholecystectomy?
Cholestyramine
Binds bile salts in colon.

Q78. Agent that reduces ammonia production by gut bacteria?
Rifaximin
Non-absorbable antibiotic.

Q79. Drug that slows colonic motility without CNS effects?
Loperamide
Does not cross BBB.

Q80. Antiemetic used in postoperative nausea and vomiting?
Ondansetron
IV route preferred perioperatively.

Q81. Antiemetic with neuroleptic properties?
Prochlorperazine
D2 blocker—used in severe nausea, vertigo.

Q82. MOA of aprepitant in emesis control?
NK1 receptor antagonist
Prevents substance P–mediated vomiting.

Q83. Which agent causes gynecomastia and galactorrhea?
Cimetidine
Antiandrogenic effects.

Q84. Antisecretory drug causing pneumonia risk in elderly?
PPIs
Alters gastric pH → bacterial overgrowth.

Q85. PPI associated with increased risk of fracture?
Yes
Due to impaired calcium absorption.

Q86. Which antiemetic is safe in pregnancy?
Doxylamine + pyridoxine
First-line for morning sickness.

Q87. Prokinetic drug used in diabetic gastroparesis?
Metoclopramide
Enhances gastric emptying.

Q88. 5-HT4 agonist used as prokinetic?
Prucalopride
For chronic constipation.

Q89. Drug that increases gastric motility without dopamine blockade?
Cisapride (withdrawn in many countries)
QT prolongation risk.

Q90. Antiemetic safe for children with gastroenteritis?
Ondansetron
Single oral dose often sufficient.

Q91. Anti–motion sickness drug with anticholinergic action?
Scopolamine
Transdermal patch.

Q92. Laxative used in opioid-induced constipation without affecting analgesia?
Methylnaltrexone
Peripheral μ-opioid receptor antagonist.

Q93. Common side effect of senna use?
Melanosis coli
Harmless pigmentation.

Q94. Which IBS drug acts on chloride channels?
Lubiprostone
Stimulates fluid secretion.

Q95. Which IBS drug acts via guanylate cyclase C activation?
Linaclotide
Increases cGMP, promotes transit.

Q96. Which drug acts both as antacid and antidiarrheal?
Bismuth subsalicylate
Useful in traveler's diarrhea.

Q97. Common antacid that causes acid rebound?
Calcium carbonate
After initial buffering.

Q98. Laxative useful in patients with hemorrhoids?
Docusate sodium
Eases defecation.

Q99. Antiemetic with risk of torsades de pointes?
Ondansetron
Especially with IV high dose.

Q100. Enzyme responsible for activation of PPIs?
Acid environment (protonation in parietal cell canaliculi)
Converts prodrug to active sulfenamide form.

Q101. Drug that increases both appetite and weight in cancer cachexia?
Megestrol acetate
A synthetic progestin with appetite stimulant properties.

Q102. Antidiarrheal contraindicated in pseudomembranous colitis?
Loperamide
Can worsen toxic megacolon in C. difficile.

Q103. Drug causing orange discoloration of body fluids and stools?
Rifampin (used in hepatic encephalopathy regimens rarely)
Harmless but alarming to patients.

Q104. Antibiotic effective against Giardia in traveler's diarrhea?
Metronidazole
Effective against anaerobes and protozoa.

Q105. Probiotic commonly used alongside antibiotics to prevent diarrhea?
Saccharomyces boulardii
Reduces risk of antibiotic-associated colitis.

Q106. MOA of dexpanthenol in GI surgery patients?
Cholinergic stimulant
Used for postoperative ileus.

Q107. Which drug used in cirrhosis reduces variceal bleeding risk?
Propranolol (non-selective β-blocker)
Decreases portal venous pressure.

Q108. Somatostatin analog used in acute variceal bleeding?
Octreotide
Reduces splanchnic blood flow.

Q109. Antiemetic avoided in Parkinson's disease?
Metoclopramide
Dopamine blockade worsens symptoms.

Q110. Bile acid used to dissolve cholesterol gallstones?
Ursodeoxycholic acid
Useful in small, radiolucent stones.

Q111. Ursodiol is contraindicated in?
Calcified or pigmented stones
Ineffective and increases recurrence.

Q112. Enzyme replacement therapy used in pancreatic insufficiency?
Pancrelipase
Improves digestion of fats and proteins.

Q113. Enzyme responsible for PPI metabolism?
CYP2C19
Genetic polymorphism affects efficacy.

Q114. Adverse effect of domperidone over long term?
QT prolongation
Monitor ECG with chronic use.

Q115. Drug that increases lower esophageal sphincter tone?
Metoclopramide
Useful in GERD.

Q116. Common side effect of PEG (polyethylene glycol)?
Bloating, flatulence
Generally well tolerated.

Q117. Purgative used for rapid colon cleansing?
Sodium phosphate
Not preferred in renal or cardiac patients.

Q118. Laxative causing phosphate nephropathy?
Sodium phosphate
Avoid in renal impairment.

Q119. Most potent PPI currently available?
Esomeprazole
S-isomer of omeprazole, higher bioavailability.

Q120. Antisecretory agent used in Zollinger-Ellison syndrome?
High-dose PPIs
H2 blockers ineffective in high gastrin states.

Q121. Antiemetic that is both a 5-HT3 and NK1 antagonist combo?
Netupitant + palonosetron
Given with dexamethasone in CINV.

Q122. GI prokinetic causing galactorrhea?
Metoclopramide
Due to dopamine blockade → ↑ prolactin.

Q123. Diarrhea in carcinoid syndrome treated with?
Octreotide
Controls flushing and secretory diarrhea.

Q124. Drug that inhibits serotonin and peptide secretion in gut tumors?
Octreotide
Somatostatin analog.

Q125. Drug causing paralytic ileus in children?
Diphenoxylate-atropine
Not safe <2 years.

Q126. GI drug with anti-inflammatory effects in ulcerative colitis?
Sulfasalazine
5-ASA + sulfapyridine.

Q127. Side effect of sulfasalazine?
Hemolysis in G6PD deficiency
Also nausea, rash, infertility.

Q128. Newer 5-ASA agent with better tolerability?
Mesalamine
Lacks sulfa moiety.

Q129. Drug of choice for Crohn's flare-up?
Corticosteroids (e.g., budesonide)
Induction agent.

Q130. Maintenance drug in IBD remission?
Azathioprine or 6-MP
Immunosuppressants.

Q131. TNF-alpha inhibitor used in IBD?
Infliximab
Effective in Crohn's and UC.

Q132. Risk of infliximab therapy?
Reactivation of TB
Screen with Mantoux or IGRA.

Q133. Biologic targeting α4β7 integrin in IBD?
Vedolizumab
Gut-selective immunosuppression.

Q134. JAK inhibitor used in ulcerative colitis?
Tofacitinib
Oral small-molecule drug.

Q135. Drug used in perianal Crohn's disease?
Infliximab
Useful in fistulizing disease.

Q136. MOA of mesalamine?
Inhibits prostaglandins and leukotrienes
Local anti-inflammatory effect.

Q137. Probiotic useful in preventing pouchitis?
VSL#3
High-potency multi-strain.

Q138. Enema form of 5-ASA is best for?
Distal ulcerative colitis
Sigmoid and rectal involvement.

Q139. Laxative useful in opioid-induced constipation in palliative care?
Naloxegol
Oral peripheral opioid antagonist.

Q140. IBS-C drug acting via guanylate cyclase-C?
Linaclotide
Enhances intestinal transit.

Q141. IBS-D treatment with non-systemic antibiotic?
Rifaximin
Modifies gut flora.

Q142. Which IBS drug is contraindicated in males?
Alosetron
Approved only for women with severe IBS-D.

Q143. Most appropriate antiemetic in pregnancy (category A/B)?
Doxylamine + pyridoxine
First-line in morning sickness.

Q144. Which gut hormone analog delays gastric emptying?
Octreotide
Also used in dumping syndrome.

Q145. Antispasmodic used in IBS?
Dicyclomine
Anticholinergic → reduces cramps.

Q146. Drug causing steatorrhea by inhibiting pancreatic lipase?
Orlistat
Used for weight loss.

Q147. Orlistat side effects?
Oily stools, flatulence, fat-soluble vitamin deficiency
Supplement vitamins A, D, E, K.

Q148. Antiemetic with extrapyramidal side effects in children?
Metoclopramide
Avoid in pediatric use unless necessary.

Q149. Drug used to prevent hepatic encephalopathy recurrence?
Rifaximin
Adjunct to lactulose.

Q150. Colon cancer prevention in IBD is improved by?
Long-term mesalamine
Has chemoprotective properties.

Q151. Antacid combination causing "acid rebound"?
Calcium carbonate + magnesium hydroxide
Calcium stimulates gastrin secretion.

Q152. Laxative preferred for anal fissures and postpartum constipation?
Stool softeners (e.g., docusate)
Minimizes straining.

Q153. GI drug that causes blue pigmentation of tongue and stool?
Bismuth subsalicylate
Harmless discoloration.

Q154. Antiemetic with highest efficacy for cisplatin-induced vomiting?
Palonosetron + dexamethasone + aprepitant
Triple antiemetic regimen.

Q155. Most common PPI side effect?
Headache and abdominal pain
Generally mild.

Q156. Anti-constipation drug causing chloride-mediated water secretion?
Lubiprostone
CIC-2 channel activator.

Q157. MOA of cholestyramine in diarrhea?
Binds bile acids
Useful in bile acid malabsorption.

Q158. OTC antidiarrheal contraindicated in children with viral enteritis?
Loperamide
Risk of ileus or toxic megacolon.

Q159. In IBS-D, 5-HT3 antagonist used is?
Alosetron
Restricted use due to ischemic colitis risk.

Q160. Drug used to prevent NSAID-induced GI bleeding in patients with CV disease?
Misoprostol (if PPI not tolerated)
Prostaglandin analog.

Q161. Prokinetic with QT-prolonging potential withdrawn in many countries?
Cisapride
Dangerous arrhythmias.

Q162. Best route of administration for ondansetron in vomiting?
IV
Rapid effect, bypasses vomiting.

Q163. Gastric cytoprotective agent that does not reduce acid secretion?
Sucralfate
Physical barrier over ulcers.

Q164. Most effective monotherapy for GERD healing?
PPIs
Heal esophagitis and reduce symptoms.

Q165. Antiemetic class useful in vertigo?
Antihistamines (e.g., promethazine)
Vestibular suppression.

Q166. Antiemetic class acting via CTZ dopamine blockade?
Phenothiazines (e.g., prochlorperazine)
Used in intractable vomiting.

Q167. Which antispasmodic has dual M3 and calcium channel blocking action?
Mebeverine
Used in IBS for cramping.

Q168. MOA of rifaximin in IBS?
Alters gut microbiota
Especially effective in bloating-predominant IBS.

Q169. Antidiarrheal that crosses BBB and causes euphoria at high doses?
Diphenoxylate
Combined with atropine to deter abuse.

Q170. Preferred antiemetic for radiotherapy-induced nausea?
5-HT3 antagonists (e.g., granisetron)
Effective in delayed emesis too.

Q171. Best time to take PPIs?
Before breakfast
Maximizes activation of proton pumps.

Q172. Probiotic helpful in antibiotic-associated diarrhea prevention?
Lactobacillus or Saccharomyces boulardii
Restores flora.

Q173. Drug causing yellow discoloration of teeth if used in children?
Tetracycline (part of H. pylori regimen)
Avoid in <8 years.

Q174. IBS-D patient with liver disease should avoid?
Alosetron
Risk of hepatic injury.

Q175. Key limitation of orlistat in obese patients?
GI side effects
Oily stools, flatulence, fecal incontinence.

Q176. Drug combination that increases the risk of C. difficile infection?
PPIs + antibiotics
Alters gut flora and pH.

Q177. Non-GI use of domperidone?
Lactation induction
Increases prolactin.

Q178. Laxative used in hepatic coma?
Lactulose
Acidifies gut to trap ammonia.

Q179. Antacid that causes "aluminum encephalopathy" in renal failure?
Aluminum hydroxide
Chronic accumulation.

Q180. GI drug that reduces cholesterol absorption and gallstone formation?
Ursodeoxycholic acid
Inhibits hepatic cholesterol secretion.

Q181. Antibiotic useful in small intestinal bacterial overgrowth (SIBO)?
Rifaximin
Minimally absorbed.

Q182. Laxative with electrolyte-free solution used before colonoscopy?
PEG (polyethylene glycol)
Non-absorbable, safe.

Q183. Major risk of sodium phosphate colon prep?
Acute phosphate nephropathy
Avoid in CKD and elderly.

Q184. IBS-D drug with opioid receptor modulation?
Eluxadoline
Mixed μ-agonist and δ-antagonist.

Q185. Warning for eluxadoline use?
Contraindicated in patients without gallbladder
Risk of pancreatitis.

Q186. Risk of metronidazole in long-term use?
Peripheral neuropathy
Monitor for paresthesia.

Q187. GI drug that may precipitate serotonin syndrome when combined with SSRIs?
Ondansetron
Both increase serotonin signaling.

Q188. PPIs may interfere with absorption of which nutrients?
Iron, B12, calcium
Due to reduced acid.

Q189. Antiemetic with dual 5-HT3 and dopamine blockade?
Metoclopramide
Acts centrally and peripherally.

Q190. Drug used to prevent NSAID-induced duodenal ulcer when PPI not tolerated?
Misoprostol
Category X in pregnancy.

Q191. Main use of glycerin suppository?
Rectal stimulant in constipation
Softens stool and induces reflex contraction.

Q192. Antacid combination causing "milk-alkali syndrome"?
Calcium + milk + alkali (e.g., bicarbonate)
Leads to hypercalcemia and alkalosis.

Q193. GI antisecretory drug that also enhances mucosal healing via VEGF?
Rebamipide
Cytoprotective (used in East Asia).

Q194. Prokinetic drug with motilin-like action?
Erythromycin
Useful in gastroparesis.

Q195. Which GI drug is used in dumping syndrome post-gastrectomy?
Octreotide
Slows gastric emptying.

Q196. Commonest side effect of rifaximin?
Bloating and flatulence
Generally well-tolerated.

Q197. Risk of gastric carcinoids with long-term hypergastrinemia?
From chronic PPI use (rare)
Seen in animal studies.

Q198. Drug used to treat gastric bezoar (pharmacologically)?
Coca-Cola lavage
Helps dissolve phytobezoars.

Q199. Drug used to treat hepatic pruritus?
Cholestyramine
Binds bile acids in gut.

Q200. Gut-selective anti-inflammatory monoclonal antibody in UC?
Vedolizumab
Targets $\alpha 4\beta 7$ integrin.

Hematologic Pharmacology

Q1. Oral anticoagulant that inhibits vitamin K epoxide reductase?
Warfarin
Interferes with synthesis of factors II, VII, IX, X.

Q2. Antidote for warfarin overdose?
Vitamin K (phytonadione)
Also FFP in life-threatening bleeding.

Q3. Warfarin monitoring is done via?
INR (International Normalized Ratio)
Target INR usually 2–3.

Q4. Heparin acts by enhancing activity of?
Antithrombin III
Inhibits thrombin and factor Xa.

Q5. Antidote for heparin toxicity?
Protamine sulfate
Binds and inactivates heparin.

Q6. Low molecular weight heparin example?
Enoxaparin
More selective for factor Xa.

Q7. LMWH vs unfractionated heparin: monitoring difference?
LMWH requires less aPTT monitoring
More predictable pharmacokinetics.

Q8. Direct oral anticoagulant (DOAC) that inhibits factor Xa?
Rivaroxaban
Also apixaban, edoxaban.

Q9. Direct thrombin inhibitor used orally?
Dabigatran
Reversibly binds thrombin.

Q10. Antidote for dabigatran?
Idarucizumab
Specific monoclonal antibody fragment.

Q11. Antidote for factor Xa inhibitors (e.g., rivaroxaban)?
Andexanet alfa
Recombinant modified factor Xa decoy.

Q12. Heparin-induced thrombocytopenia (HIT) is mediated by?
IgG antibodies against heparin-PF4 complex
Activates platelets.

Q13. Drug used in HIT instead of heparin?
Argatroban
Direct thrombin inhibitor.

Q14. Antiplatelet drug that irreversibly inhibits COX-1?
Aspirin
Blocks thromboxane A_2 production.

Q15. Platelet aggregation test affected by aspirin?
Bleeding time
Not PT or aPTT.

Q16. ADP receptor blocker used in dual antiplatelet therapy?
Clopidogrel
Prodrug; inhibits P2Y12 receptor.

Q17. Clopidogrel activation depends on which enzyme?
CYP2C19
Poor metabolizers have reduced effect.

Q18. Newer P2Y12 inhibitors with faster action?
Prasugrel, ticagrelor
More consistent platelet inhibition.

Q19. Antiplatelet with reversible P2Y12 inhibition?
Ticagrelor
Direct-acting, not a prodrug.

Q20. GPIIb/IIIa receptor inhibitor used in PCI?
Abciximab
Prevents fibrinogen binding.

Q21. Abciximab is derived from?
Monoclonal antibody
Chimeric Fab fragment.

Q22. Drug that inhibits phosphodiesterase and increases cAMP in platelets?
Dipyridamole
Weak antiplatelet + vasodilator.

Q23. Use of cilostazol in peripheral artery disease?
Improves claudication symptoms
PDE-3 inhibitor with antiplatelet effect.

Q24. Fibrinolytic agent used in acute stroke or MI?
Alteplase (tPA)
Converts plasminogen to plasmin.

Q25. Antidote for tPA overdose or bleeding?
Aminocaproic acid or tranexamic acid
Inhibit fibrinolysis.

Q26. Drug of choice for pulmonary embolism in hemodynamically unstable patients?
Alteplase
Thrombolytic therapy.

Q27. Oral iron supplement commonly used in anemia?
Ferrous sulfate
20% elemental iron.

Q28. Side effects of oral iron?
GI upset, constipation, black stools
Dose-related.

Q29. Drug that enhances iron absorption?
Ascorbic acid (vitamin C)
Reduces ferric to ferrous form.

Q30. Parenteral iron preparation with least risk of anaphylaxis?
Iron sucrose
Safer than iron dextran.

Q31. Erythropoietin analog used in CKD anemia?
Epoetin alfa
Stimulates erythropoiesis.

Q32. Risk of using erythropoietin in high doses?
Hypertension, thromboembolism
Use lowest effective dose.

Q33. Hematopoietic agent used in chemotherapy-induced neutropenia?
Filgrastim (G-CSF)
Stimulates neutrophil production.

Q34. Pegfilgrastim advantage over filgrastim?
Longer half-life
Once-per-cycle dosing.

Q35. GM-CSF analog used in bone marrow recovery?
Sargramostim
Stimulates granulocytes + macrophages.

Q36. Oral iron chelator used in thalassemia?
Deferasirox
Once-daily dosing.

Q37. Parenteral iron chelator used in iron overload?
Deferoxamine
Binds ferric iron.

Q38. Vitamin used to reverse methotrexate-induced anemia?
Folinic acid (leucovorin)
Rescues normal cells.

Q39. Drug causing folate deficiency anemia?
Phenytoin, methotrexate, TMP-SMX
Antifolate effect.

Q40. Drug causing macrocytic anemia with neurologic signs?
Nitrous oxide abuse
Inactivates vitamin B12.

Q41. IM vitamin B12 preparation?
Hydroxocobalamin
Longer half-life than cyanocobalamin.

Q42. Common anemia in chronic inflammation?
Anemia of chronic disease
Due to hepcidin-mediated iron restriction.

Q43. Drug causing aplastic anemia as rare but serious side effect?
Chloramphenicol
Irreversible and dose-independent.

Q44. Drug causing dose-dependent megaloblastic anemia?
Azathioprine
Suppresses bone marrow.

Q45. Preferred iron preparation in pregnancy?
Ferrous sulfate or fumarate
Well tolerated, inexpensive.

Q46. Enzyme inhibited by hydroxyurea in sickle cell disease?
Ribonucleotide reductase
Increases HbF.

Q47. MOA of hydroxyurea in sickle cell disease?
Increases fetal hemoglobin (HbF)
Reduces sickling.

Q48. Drug used to reduce bleeding in hemophilia or surgery?
Tranexamic acid
Antifibrinolytic.

Q49. Antiplatelet drug safe in aspirin allergy?
Clopidogrel
Alternative for secondary prevention.

Q50. Drug used to reverse NOACs (e.g., apixaban, rivaroxaban)?
Andexanet alfa
Factor Xa decoy protein.

Q51. Recombinant factor VIII is used in?
Hemophilia A
Replace deficient factor VIII.

Q52. Recombinant factor IX is used in?
Hemophilia B
Also called Christmas disease.

Q53. Drug used to prevent bleeding in von Willebrand disease?
Desmopressin (DDAVP)
Releases vWF and factor VIII.

Q54. Desmopressin is ineffective in which vWD type?
Type 3 vWD
Severe deficiency – needs factor replacement.

Q55. Drug used to prevent thrombosis in atrial fibrillation?
Apixaban or warfarin
Reduces stroke risk.

Q56. Long-term anticoagulant in mechanical heart valves?
Warfarin
INR goal 2.5–3.5 (higher than usual).

Q57. Drug interaction: warfarin effect increased by?
Amiodarone, metronidazole
CYP inhibition ↑ INR.

Q58. Warfarin effect decreased by?
Rifampin, carbamazepine
CYP induction ↓ INR.

Q59. LMWH advantage over UFH?
Better bioavailability, less HIT
No aPTT monitoring usually needed.

Q60. Anticoagulant safe in pregnancy?
Heparin
Does not cross placenta.

Q61. Anticoagulant contraindicated in pregnancy?
Warfarin
Teratogenic – causes fetal bleeding, bone defects.

Q62. Bleeding disorder due to platelet function defect, not number?
Glanzmann thrombasthenia
GPIIb/IIIa defect.

Q63. Platelet receptor blocked by abciximab?
GPIIb/IIIa
Prevents fibrinogen-mediated aggregation.

Q64. Lab parameter elevated in vitamin K deficiency?
PT (prothrombin time)
Affects factors II, VII, IX, X.

Q65. Drug-induced lupus with anti-histone antibodies and anemia?
Hydralazine
May also cause hemolysis.

Q66. Preferred anticoagulant in cancer-associated thrombosis?
LMWH (e.g., enoxaparin)
DOACs are alternative options now.

Q67. Drug used to treat thrombotic thrombocytopenic purpura (TTP)?
Plasma exchange + steroids
Caplacizumab (anti-vWF) also used.

Q68. Most common cause of megaloblastic anemia?
Vitamin B12 or folate deficiency
Macrocytosis with hypersegmented neutrophils.

Q69. Drug that may cause macrocytic anemia without neurologic symptoms?
Methotrexate
Pure folate deficiency.

Q70. Drug class causing agranulocytosis?
Antithyroid drugs (e.g., PTU), clozapine
Sudden and severe neutropenia.

Q71. Iron chelator safe in thalassemia major?
Deferasirox
Oral option for iron overload.

Q72. Hematologic side effect of linezolid?
Bone marrow suppression
Especially thrombocytopenia.

Q73. Enzyme deficiency causing hemolytic anemia with oxidant drugs?
G6PD deficiency
Triggered by sulfa, fava beans, etc.

Q74. Drug used to increase platelet count in ITP?
Eltrombopag
TPO receptor agonist.

Q75. Anti-CD20 monoclonal antibody used in ITP?
Rituximab
Destroys B cells producing autoantibodies.

Q76. Drug causing dose-dependent thrombocytopenia?
Carboplatin, paclitaxel
Common chemo-related toxicity.

Q77. Drug that increases risk of arterial thrombosis in cancer?
Thalidomide, lenalidomide
Need thromboprophylaxis.

Q78. Anticoagulant requiring renal dose adjustment?
Dabigatran, rivaroxaban
Excreted by kidneys.

Q79. Drug with highest bleeding risk among anticoagulants?
Warfarin (especially high INR)
Requires regular monitoring.

Q80. Drug with fastest onset among oral anticoagulants?
Apixaban and rivaroxaban
Peak action within hours.

Q81. Warfarin-induced skin necrosis is due to?
Protein C depletion
Occurs early in therapy.

Q82. Prothrombin complex concentrate (PCC) contains?
Factors II, VII, IX, X
Rapid INR reversal.

Q83. Fibrinolytic with longest half-life?
Tenecteplase
Single bolus thrombolysis in MI.

Q84. Agent used to reduce bleeding in dental procedures in hemophilia?
Tranexamic acid mouthwash
Topical antifibrinolytic.

Q85. Drug used to reduce transfusion needs in uremic bleeding?
Desmopressin
Enhances platelet adhesion via vWF.

Q86. Drug that mimics action of erythropoietin but is orally active?
Roxadustat (experimental)
HIF prolyl hydroxylase inhibitor.

Q87. Methotrexate toxicity reversed by?
Leucovorin (folinic acid)
"Rescue" therapy.

Q88. Bone marrow failure from chemotherapy reversed by?
Filgrastim, epoetin, thrombopoietin agonists
Depending on lineage affected.

Q89. Preferred anticoagulant in massive PE with shock?
Unfractionated heparin IV
Rapid onset, titratable.

Q90. Drug that reduces hemolysis in paroxysmal nocturnal hemoglobinuria (PNH)?
Eculizumab
C5 complement inhibitor.

Q91. Heparin side effect seen with long-term use?
Osteoporosis
Especially with high-dose UFH.

Q92. Iron preparation with black-box warning for anaphylaxis?
Iron dextran
Test dose required.

Q93. Vitamin required for heme synthesis?
Vitamin B6 (pyridoxine)
Needed in sideroblastic anemia.

Q94. Drug causing sideroblastic anemia by B6 depletion?
Isoniazid
Supplement pyridoxine.

Q95. Drug with both immunosuppressive and anti-anemia effect in MDS?
Lenalidomide
Also used in 5q- syndrome.

Q96. Risk of erythropoietin-stimulating agents in cancer patients?
Thromboembolism and tumor progression
Use cautiously.

Q97. Baseline test before starting epoetin?
Iron studies
Functional iron deficiency is common.

Q98. Which oral anticoagulant is contraindicated in valvular AF?
DOACs (e.g., apixaban, rivaroxaban)
Use warfarin.

Q99. MOA of fondaparinux?
Factor Xa inhibition via antithrombin
No effect on thrombin.

Q100. Half-life of warfarin is prolonged in which genetic mutation?
CYP2C9 2 or 3
Slow metabolism → higher bleeding risk.

Q101. Which iron formulation is most likely to cause hypotension on IV administration?
Iron dextran
Risk of anaphylaxis and hypotension—test dose mandatory.

Q102. Key lab finding in warfarin overdose?
Prolonged PT/INR
Affects extrinsic pathway.

Q103. Antidote for fibrinolytic drug toxicity?
Tranexamic acid
Inhibits plasminogen activation.

Q104. Which blood product contains all clotting factors including fibrinogen?
Fresh frozen plasma (FFP)
Used in active bleeding with coagulopathy.

Q105. First coagulation factor depleted by warfarin therapy?
Factor VII
Shortest half-life.

Q106. In DIC, which pharmacological treatment may be considered?
Cryoprecipitate, platelets, FFP
Supportive care + treat cause.

Q107. Which anemia-causing drug inhibits DNA synthesis via DHFR inhibition?

Methotrexate
Leads to megaloblastic anemia.

Q108. In B12 deficiency anemia, methylmalonic acid levels are?
Increased
Differentiates from folate deficiency.

Q109. Drug-induced hemolysis is most often associated with?
G6PD deficiency
Triggered by sulfa, antimalarials.

Q110. Which hemostatic drug is a synthetic analog of lysine?
Tranexamic acid
Antifibrinolytic.

Q111. MOA of eculizumab?
C5 complement inhibition
Used in PNH and atypical HUS.

Q112. Which anticoagulant does not affect aPTT or PT?
Fondaparinux
Selectively inhibits factor Xa.

Q113. Drug of choice in stroke prevention in AF patients with valvular heart disease?
Warfarin
DOACs not approved in valvular AF.

Q114. Which RBC growth factor is used in anemia of chronic kidney disease?
Erythropoietin (EPO) analogs
Eg: epoetin alfa, darbepoetin.

Q115. Major ADR of erythropoietin analogs?
Hypertension
Due to rapid rise in RBC mass.

Q116. Which synthetic EPO has the longest half-life?
Darbepoetin alfa
Modified glycosylation increases duration.

Q117. Which drug is a thrombopoietin receptor agonist?
Eltrombopag
Used in chronic ITP and aplastic anemia.

Q118. Anticoagulant that causes purple toe syndrome?

Warfarin

Due to cholesterol microembolism.

Q119. Which factor is not vitamin K dependent?

Factor V

II, VII, IX, X are vitamin K dependent.

Q120. Which agent increases gamma-globin synthesis in sickle cell disease?

Hydroxyurea

Increases HbF.

Q121. Which anti-inflammatory drug reduces platelet aggregation at low dose?

Aspirin

Irreversibly inhibits COX-1.

Q122. Aspirin resistance is due to polymorphism in?

COX-1 gene

Rare but significant in CV patients.

Q123. Most common ADR of ticlopidine?

Neutropenia

Replaced by safer alternatives.

Q124. Difference between ticagrelor and clopidogrel?

Ticagrelor is reversible and not a prodrug

Faster onset.

Q125. Which lab test is best to monitor LMWH effect?

Anti-factor Xa level

aPTT not reliable.

Q126. Which iron chelator is safe orally and for long-term use?

Deferasirox

Once daily dosing.

Q127. Which enzyme deficiency causes porphyria with photosensitivity?

Uroporphyrinogen decarboxylase

Porphyria cutanea tarda.

Q128. Drug that may trigger acute intermittent porphyria attack?

Barbiturates

Induce ALA synthase.

Q129. Drug that treats acute porphyria attack by negative feedback?
Hemin
Suppresses ALA synthase.

Q130. Primary drug for iron-deficiency anemia?
Ferrous sulfate
Cost-effective, standard dose.

Q131. Drug that increases absorption of oral iron?
Ascorbic acid
Acidifies GI tract.

Q132. Chelator used for aluminum toxicity in dialysis?
Deferoxamine
Binds aluminum and iron.

Q133. Drug used to reduce platelet activation in stent placement?
Clopidogrel
P2Y12 blocker.

Q134. Most serious side effect of tPA?
Intracranial hemorrhage
Risk ↑ in elderly or HTN.

Q135. Drug used for bleeding in menorrhagia?
Tranexamic acid
Stabilizes clot.

Q136. Which oral drug mimics endogenous thrombopoietin?
Romiplostim (SC) or eltrombopag (oral)
Activates TPO receptor.

Q137. Drug that improves fetal hemoglobin production?
Hydroxyurea
Also cytotoxic.

Q138. Which antiplatelet is a reversible non-competitive P2Y12 inhibitor?
Ticagrelor
Not dependent on liver metabolism.

Q139. Clopidogrel resistance occurs due to mutation in?
CYP2C19
Reduces activation.

Q140. Anticoagulant causing osteoporosis on long-term use?
Heparin
Due to bone resorption.

Q141. Drug used in factor VIII inhibitor–positive hemophilia A?
Emicizumab
Bispecific antibody bridging factors IXa and X.

Q142. Which lab test is falsely prolonged in lupus anticoagulant?
aPTT
Despite hypercoagulable state.

Q143. Drug used for HIT with normal renal function?
Argatroban
Monitored by aPTT.

Q144. Which anticoagulant increases antithrombin activity?
Heparin
Rapid action.

Q145. Fibrinolytic used in ischemic stroke within 4.5 hours?
Alteplase (tPA)
Time-sensitive.

Q146. Which drug inhibits thrombin directly?
Dabigatran
Oral DTI.

Q147. Which anti-platelet drug inhibits adenosine reuptake?
Dipyridamole
↑ cAMP, inhibits aggregation.

Q148. Genetic polymorphism causing resistance to clopidogrel?
CYP2C19 loss-of-function
Poor responders.

Q149. Anticoagulant that inhibits both free and clot-bound thrombin?
Dabigatran
Direct thrombin inhibitor.

Q150. Factor X inhibitor with oral route and renal excretion?
Rivaroxaban
Fixed dose, no routine monitoring.

Q151. Heparin's anticoagulant activity is measured by?
aPTT
Prolonged with unfractionated heparin.

Q152. Warfarin therapy initially causes hypercoagulability due to?
Protein C depletion
Short half-life compared to clotting factors.

Q153. Anticoagulant contraindicated with spinal/epidural anesthesia?
LMWH
Risk of spinal hematoma.

Q154. Preferred agent for prevention of thromboembolism in orthopedic surgery?
LMWH
Started 12–24 hrs post-op.

Q155. Hematologic side effect of valproic acid?
Thrombocytopenia
Also impairs platelet function.

Q156. Anemia caused by lead poisoning is?
Microcytic, hypochromic
Also basophilic stippling.

Q157. Enzyme inhibited by lead in heme synthesis?
Ferrochelatase and ALA dehydratase
Leads to anemia and neurotoxicity.

Q158. Treatment for lead poisoning in adults?
EDTA or dimercaprol
Chelation therapy.

Q159. DOC for iron poisoning?
Deferoxamine
Chelates ferric iron.

Q160. Best marker for response to iron therapy?
Reticulocyte count
Increases within a week.

Q161. Drug causing macrocytic anemia without neuro signs?
Methotrexate
Due to folate deficiency.

Q162. Drug-induced aplastic anemia is most associated with?
Chloramphenicol
Rare but fatal.

Q163. Drug that causes hemolytic anemia in cold temperatures?
Methyldopa
Autoimmune hemolysis.

Q164. In TTP, plasma exchange removes?
Autoantibodies to ADAMTS13
Also replaces functional enzyme.

Q165. Treatment for B12 deficiency anemia?
Hydroxocobalamin IM
Preferred over cyanocobalamin.

Q166. Hemostatic agent used in dental extraction in hemophilia patients?
Tranexamic acid
Topical application.

Q167. Use of desmopressin in uremic bleeding?
Improves platelet function
Temporarily increases vWF.

Q168. Which medication can be used to treat hemophilia A with inhibitors?
Emicizumab
Factor VIII mimetic antibody.

Q169. Reversal agent for factor Xa inhibitors (e.g. apixaban)?
Andexanet alfa
Decoy receptor.

Q170. Thrombopoietin receptor agonist for aplastic anemia?
Eltrombopag
Stimulates hematopoietic stem cells.

Q171. Chemo drug causing delayed thrombocytopenia?
Carboplatin
Often dose-limiting.

Q172. Romiplostim is administered via which route?
Subcutaneous
Used in chronic ITP.

Q173. Monitoring required for eltrombopag therapy?
LFTs
Risk of hepatotoxicity.

Q174. Emicizumab acts by bridging which factors?
IXa and X
Mimics factor VIII.

Q175. RBC abnormality seen with pyridoxine deficiency?
Sideroblastic anemia
Due to impaired heme synthesis.

Q176. Drug that increases HbF in sickle cell patients?
Hydroxyurea
Reduces vaso-occlusive crises.

Q177. Drug causing B12 deficiency by impairing absorption?
Metformin
Especially with long-term use.

Q178. Which class of drugs increases bleeding time but not PT or aPTT?
Antiplatelets
Eg: aspirin, clopidogrel.

Q179. Drug class that prolongs both PT and aPTT?
Direct thrombin inhibitors
Eg: dabigatran, argatroban.

Q180. Drug-induced eosinophilia is commonly seen with?
Minocycline, phenytoin
Often mild.

Q181. Coagulopathy in DIC is best treated with?
FFP + platelet transfusion
Corrects clotting factor deficits.

Q182. Drug-induced pancytopenia is most associated with?
Chemotherapy agents
Eg: busulfan, cyclophosphamide.

Q183. Pseudo-thrombocytopenia is due to?
Platelet clumping in EDTA tubes
Use citrate tubes instead.

Q184. Drug that increases bleeding risk if combined with NSAIDs?
SSRIs
Impair platelet aggregation.

Q185. MOA of fondaparinux?
Indirect Xa inhibitor via antithrombin
No thrombin inhibition.

Q186. Iron chelator contraindicated in renal failure?
Deferasirox
Risk of nephrotoxicity.

Q187. Which drug reduces incidence of febrile neutropenia in chemo?
Filgrastim
Stimulates neutrophil recovery.

Q188. Most serious adverse effect of G-CSF therapy?
Splenic rupture (rare)
Monitor for LUQ pain.

Q189. Darbepoetin is preferred over epoetin alfa due to?
Longer half-life
Less frequent dosing.

Q190. Contraindication to erythropoietin therapy?
Uncontrolled hypertension
Can worsen BP.

Q191. Sickle cell anemia crisis prevention drug?
Hydroxyurea
Increases HbF.

Q192. Most common side effect of ferrous sulfate?
Constipation
GI upset common.

Q193. Anticoagulant that binds directly to thrombin?
Dabigatran
Oral DTI.

Q194. Anticoagulant with lowest HIT risk?
Fondaparinux
Synthetic, no heparin core.

Q195. Fibrinolytic agent preferred for massive PE?
Alteplase
Systemic thrombolysis.

Q196. Initial bridge therapy when starting warfarin?
Heparin
Prevents protein C depletion thrombosis.

Q197. Anemia of chronic disease is associated with high levels of?
Hepcidin
Blocks iron absorption and release.

Q198. Major limitation of clopidogrel use?
Genetic variability (CYP2C19 polymorphism)
Affects efficacy.

Q199. Reversal of warfarin in emergency bleeding includes?
PCC + Vitamin K
Rapid INR correction.

Q200. Platelet function in uremia can be improved by?
Desmopressin
Increases vWF release.

Renal Pharmacology

Q1. Site of action of loop diuretics?
Thick ascending limb of loop of Henle
Inhibit $Na^+/K^+/2Cl^-$ cotransporter.

Q2. Example of a loop diuretic?
Furosemide
Others: torsemide, bumetanide.

Q3. Adverse effect of loop diuretics?
Hypokalemia, ototoxicity
Also causes hypocalcemia.

Q4. Which diuretic causes hypercalcemia?
Thiazide diuretics
Reduce urinary calcium excretion.

Q5. Site of action of thiazides?
Distal convoluted tubule
Inhibit Na^+/Cl^- symporter.

Q6. Example of a thiazide diuretic?
Hydrochlorothiazide
Also indapamide, chlorthalidone.

Q7. Electrolyte abnormality with thiazide use?
Hyponatremia, hypokalemia, hyperuricemia
May cause gout flare.

Q8. Potassium-sparing diuretics act on?
Collecting duct
Inhibit Na^+ channels or aldosterone receptors.

Q9. Example of aldosterone antagonist?
Spironolactone
Others: eplerenone.

Q10. Spironolactone can cause which endocrine side effect?
Gynecomastia
Due to anti-androgen effect.

Q11. Eplerenone is preferred over spironolactone because?
Less gynecomastia
More selective aldosterone antagonist.

Q12. Osmotic diuretic used in cerebral edema?
Mannitol
Increases plasma osmolarity.

Q13. Contraindication for mannitol?
Heart failure
May cause pulmonary edema.

Q14. Diuretic causing metabolic alkalosis?
Loop and thiazide diuretics
Due to H^+ loss.

Q15. Diuretic causing metabolic acidosis?
Acetazolamide
Carbonic anhydrase inhibitor.

Q16. Acetazolamide acts on which segment?
Proximal tubule
Inhibits HCO_3^- reabsorption.

Q17. Clinical use of acetazolamide besides diuresis?
Glaucoma, altitude sickness, metabolic alkalosis
Induces mild acidosis.

Q18. Major electrolyte loss with acetazolamide?
Bicarbonate
Leads to metabolic acidosis.

Q19. Drug that reduces intraocular pressure rapidly?
Acetazolamide
Used in acute angle-closure glaucoma.

Q20. Diuretic preferred in nephrolithiasis due to hypercalciuria?
Thiazides
Promote calcium reabsorption.

Q21. Diuretic used in lithium-induced diabetes insipidus?
Amiloride
Blocks ENaC and lithium entry.

Q22. Most potent class of diuretics?
Loop diuretics
High ceiling effect.

Q23. Diuretic contraindicated in sulfa allergy?
Furosemide, hydrochlorothiazide
Ethacrynic acid is safe alternative.

Q24. Diuretic that may worsen gout?
Thiazides and loop diuretics
Increase uric acid reabsorption.

Q25. Diuretic safe in hypercalcemia?
Furosemide
Promotes calcium excretion.

Q26. Drugs that reduce proteinuria in CKD?
ACE inhibitors
Decrease intraglomerular pressure.

Q27. ACE inhibitors act by inhibiting?
Angiotensin-converting enzyme
↓ Ang II and aldosterone.

Q28. ACE inhibitor side effects?
Cough, hyperkalemia, angioedema
Cough due to bradykinin.

Q29. ARB example?
Losartan
Blocks AT1 receptor directly.

Q30. ARBs are preferred over ACE inhibitors when?
Cough or angioedema with ACEi
Similar renal protection.

Q31. Direct renin inhibitor?
Aliskiren
↓ Plasma renin activity.

Q32. NSAIDs reduce diuretic efficacy by?
Constricting afferent arteriole
↓ GFR and natriuresis.

Q33. Drug that dilates the efferent arteriole?
ACE inhibitors
↓ Glomerular pressure.

Q34. Drug that constricts afferent arteriole?
NSAIDs
↓ Prostaglandin-mediated dilation.

Q35. Hyperkalemia-prone combination?
ACEi + spironolactone
Monitor serum potassium.

Q36. Drug causing nephrogenic diabetes insipidus?
Lithium
Interferes with ADH action.

Q37. Drug used to treat central diabetes insipidus?
Desmopressin
Synthetic ADH analog.

Q38. Drug causing interstitial nephritis?
Methicillin, NSAIDs
Presents with fever, eosinophilia.

Q39. Antibiotic causing acute tubular necrosis (ATN)?
Aminoglycosides
Dose-related nephrotoxicity.

Q40. Electrolyte imbalance seen with amphotericin B?
Hypokalemia and hypomagnesemia
Due to renal tubular damage.

Q41. Drug used to alkalinize urine in rhabdomyolysis?
Sodium bicarbonate
Prevents myoglobin nephrotoxicity.

Q42. Contrast-induced nephropathy prevention?
IV hydration ± N-acetylcysteine
Avoid NSAIDs.

Q43. Diuretic causing ototoxicity?
Furosemide
Especially IV high doses.

Q44. Drug used in hepatorenal syndrome?
Midodrine + octreotide + albumin
Improve renal perfusion.

Q45. SGLT2 inhibitors reduce progression of?
Diabetic nephropathy
Eg: empagliflozin, dapagliflozin.

Q46. MOA of SGLT2 inhibitors?
Inhibit glucose reabsorption in PCT
Induce glucosuria and natriuresis.

Q47. SGLT2 inhibitors adverse effects?
UTIs, genital mycotic infections
Due to glycosuria.

Q48. Diuretic used in acute pulmonary edema?
Furosemide (IV)
Rapid venodilation and diuresis.

Q49. Drug class improving heart and kidney outcomes in diabetics?
SGLT2 inhibitors
Cardiorenal protection.

Q50. Antidiuretic hormone antagonist used in SIADH?
Tolvaptan
V2 receptor antagonist.

Q51. Loop diuretic with the longest duration of action?
Torsemide
Longer half-life than furosemide.

Q52. Drug used to prevent cisplatin-induced nephrotoxicity?
Amifostine
Cytoprotective agent.

Q53. Key feature of NSAID-induced AKI?
Reduced prostaglandins → afferent arteriole constriction
↓ GFR.

Q54. Best initial management for contrast-induced nephropathy?
IV hydration with normal saline
Prevents tubular injury.

Q55. Drug used to alkalinize urine in tumor lysis syndrome?
Sodium bicarbonate
Prevents uric acid crystallization.

Q56. Drug causing papillary necrosis in kidneys?
NSAIDs
Chronic use—especially in diabetics.

Q57. Nephrotoxic effect of cyclosporine?
Dose-dependent vasoconstriction
Also causes hypertension.

Q58. Immunosuppressant causing hyperuricemia and nephrotoxicity?
Tacrolimus
Similar to cyclosporine.

Q59. Which antidiabetic class causes osmotic diuresis?
SGLT2 inhibitors (e.g., empagliflozin)
Glucosuria-induced water loss.

Q60. Renal effect of mannitol?
Osmotic diuretic → ↑ urine output
Risk of volume overload if not cleared.

Q61. Diuretic that improves mortality in heart failure?
Spironolactone
Aldosterone antagonist benefit.

Q62. ACE inhibitors reduce proteinuria by?
Efferent arteriole dilation
Lowers glomerular pressure.

Q63. Diuretic causing hypokalemic metabolic alkalosis?
Loop or thiazide diuretics
Due to volume loss and RAAS activation.

Q64. Most nephrotoxic aminoglycoside?
Gentamicin
Accumulates in proximal tubule.

Q65. Diuretic combination causing profound hypokalemia?
Loop + thiazide
Add K^+-sparing to prevent.

Q66. Aldosterone antagonist selective for mineralocorticoid receptor?
Eplerenone
Less antiandrogenic than spironolactone.

Q67. Diuretic contraindicated in hyperkalemia?
Spironolactone, amiloride
May worsen K^+ levels.

Q68. Renal effect of vancomycin?
Acute tubular necrosis
Dose-related.

Q69. Drug used to prevent uric acid nephropathy in tumor lysis syndrome?
Rasburicase
Converts uric acid to allantoin.

Q70. Antifungal with high nephrotoxicity?
Amphotericin B
Causes tubular damage and vasoconstriction.

Q71. Diuretic with sulfonamide structure?
All except ethacrynic acid
Caution in sulfa allergy.

Q72. Which antihypertensive causes hyperkalemia especially in CKD?
ACE inhibitors or ARBs
Monitor K^+ levels.

Q73. Non-dihydropyridine CCB causing minimal renal protection?
Verapamil
Less effective than ACEi in proteinuria.

Q74. Drug increasing serum creatinine without actual nephrotoxicity?
Cimetidine or trimethoprim
Compete for creatinine secretion.

Q75. Agent that can falsely elevate creatinine levels in lab tests?
Cefoxitin
Interferes with assay.

Q76. Diuretic that may worsen gout?
Thiazides
↑ Uric acid reabsorption.

Q77. Mechanism of edema in nephrotic syndrome?
Hypoalbuminemia + RAAS activation
Treat with diuretics.

Q78. Drug-induced nephrolithiasis is associated with?
Indinavir (HIV drug), topiramate
Crystalluria.

Q79. Most nephrotoxic antiviral in transplant patients?
Acyclovir (IV)
Dose adjust in renal failure.

Q80. Diuretic most effective at removing sodium?
Loop diuretics
Act upstream of macula densa.

Q81. First-line for BP control in CKD with proteinuria?
ACE inhibitors
Delay progression.

Q82. Aldosterone antagonist used in resistant hypertension?
Spironolactone
Particularly useful in hyperaldosteronism.

Q83. Drug that mimics nephrogenic DI effect?
Lithium
Blocks aquaporin-2.

Q84. Vaptans can cause?
Rapid correction of sodium
Risk of osmotic demyelination.

Q85. Diuretic choice in cirrhosis with ascites?
Spironolactone ± furosemide
Corrects secondary hyperaldosteronism.

Q86. Thiazide diuretic with longer half-life and less metabolic effects?
Chlorthalidone
Preferred for HTN.

Q87. Antifungal safe in renal dysfunction?
Fluconazole
Dose adjust but less nephrotoxic.

Q88. Drug with narrow therapeutic window, requires renal monitoring?
Digoxin
Risk of toxicity in CKD.

Q89. SGLT2 inhibitor renal benefits include?
↓ Proteinuria, ↓ GFR decline
Also CV protection.

Q90. MOA of sodium polystyrene sulfonate?
Cation exchange resin
Binds K^+ in colon.

Q91. Drug used to treat hyperphosphatemia in CKD?
Sevelamer
Phosphate binder.

Q92. Iron-based phosphate binder?
Ferric citrate
Lowers P and replenishes iron.

Q93. Drug causing renal magnesium wasting?
Cisplatin
Hypomagnesemia is common.

Q94. Renal mechanism of NSAID nephrotoxicity?
Inhibit prostaglandin synthesis → vasoconstriction
Especially in pre-renal states.

Q95. Diuretic that causes tinnitus in high doses?
Furosemide
Ototoxicity risk.

Q96. Antiviral requiring prehydration due to nephrotoxicity?
Acyclovir
Prevent crystal precipitation.

Q97. Antibiotic associated with Fanconi syndrome?
Tenofovir
Proximal tubular dysfunction.

Q98. Drug class that increases uric acid excretion?
Uricosurics (e.g., probenecid)
Risk of uric acid stones.

Q99. Renal drug class contraindicated in hypovolemia?
ACE inhibitors
Risk of AKI.

Q100. Potassium binder safe in chronic hyperkalemia?
Patiromer
Delayed action, oral.

Q101. Diuretic class contraindicated in anuria?
Thiazides
Ineffective when GFR is very low.

Q102. Nephrotoxic antibiotic with both tubular and glomerular effects?
Amphotericin B
Causes vasoconstriction + tubular damage.

Q103. Agent used to treat tumor lysis syndrome hyperuricemia?
Rasburicase
Converts uric acid to allantoin.

Q104. NSAID effect on renal prostaglandins leads to?
Afferent arteriole vasoconstriction
↓ GFR, especially in hypovolemia.

Q105. Diuretic that may cause photosensitivity?
Thiazides
Rare, but known adverse effect.

Q106. Long-term loop diuretic use may lead to?
Secondary hyperaldosteronism
Due to volume depletion.

Q107. Drug causing hyperkalemia and metabolic acidosis?
Spironolactone
Aldosterone antagonism.

Q108. Antihypertensive that reduces intraglomerular pressure?
ACE inhibitors
Dilation of efferent arteriole.

Q109. Thiazide-induced glucose intolerance mechanism?
Hypokalemia impairs insulin release
Can worsen glycemic control.

Q110. Antiviral causing obstructive nephropathy?
Acyclovir (IV)
Crystals in renal tubules.

Q111. Renal complication of methotrexate?
Crystalluria
Hydration helps prevent.

Q112. Electrolyte imbalance due to mannitol overuse?
Hypernatremia
From free water loss.

Q113. Hypomagnesemia is seen with chronic use of?
Loop diuretics
May also cause hypocalcemia.

Q114. Diuretic that may unmask latent diabetes insipidus?
Lithium
Induces nephrogenic DI.

Q115. Renal drug that should be avoided with metformin in CKD?
Contrast media
↑ Risk of lactic acidosis.

Q116. Diuretic useful in idiopathic hypercalciuria?
Thiazides
↓ Calcium excretion.

Q117. Diuretic class promoting bicarbonate excretion?
Carbonic anhydrase inhibitors
Causes metabolic acidosis.

Q118. Nephrotoxic drug that also causes anemia due to renal injury?
Cisplatin
Affects EPO-producing cells.

Q119. SGLT2 inhibitors lead to mild diuresis by?
Blocking glucose reabsorption
Osmotic effect.

Q120. Which phosphate binder is not calcium-based?
Sevelamer
Non-absorbable polymer.

Q121. Drug that improves renal outcomes in diabetics even without proteinuria?

SGLT2 inhibitors
Eg: empagliflozin, dapagliflozin.

Q122. Drug class reducing cardiovascular mortality in CKD?

SGLT2 inhibitors
Multiple protective effects.

Q123. Class of diuretics that increase urine calcium?

Loop diuretics
Opposite of thiazides.

Q124. Osmotic diuretic effect on serum potassium?

May cause hyperkalemia
Due to volume contraction.

Q125. Drug used for ADPKD slowing progression?

Tolvaptan
V2 receptor antagonist.

Q126. Risk of rapid sodium correction with vaptans?

Osmotic demyelination syndrome
Monitor closely.

Q127. Antihypertensive contraindicated in bilateral RAS?

ACE inhibitors
May cause acute renal failure.

Q128. Best agent to manage uric acid nephropathy in TLS?

Rasburicase
More effective than allopurinol.

Q129. Drug that decreases serum uric acid AND provides iron?

Ferric citrate
Dual benefit in CKD.

Q130. Uremia-related platelet dysfunction managed by?

Desmopressin
Increases vWF levels.

Q131. Drug used to prevent NSAID-induced nephropathy?
Misoprostol
Prostaglandin analog.

Q132. Preferred contrast agent in renal impairment?
Iso-osmolar, non-ionic contrast
Eg: iodixanol.

Q133. Renal drug with narrow therapeutic index and peak-trough monitoring?
Digoxin
Renally excreted—caution in CKD.

Q134. Antiviral needing dose adjustment in renal failure?
Acyclovir
Prevent toxicity.

Q135. Antifungal with lowest renal risk?
Fluconazole
Adjust dose but minimal nephrotoxicity.

Q136. Gout drug used in renal impairment?
Febuxostat
Safer than allopurinol in CKD.

Q137. Loop diuretic causing the most hearing loss risk?
Ethacrynic acid
Ototoxicity worse than furosemide.

Q138. Electrolyte effect of ACE inhibitors?
Hyperkalemia
Especially in CKD, diabetes.

Q139. Thiazide + ACE inhibitor combination advantage?
ACEi corrects thiazide-induced hypokalemia
Better BP control.

Q140. Nephrotoxic combination to avoid?
ACE inhibitor + NSAID + diuretic
"Triple whammy" → AKI.

Q141. MOA of patiromer in hyperkalemia?
Binds K^+ in colon
Promotes fecal K^+ excretion.

Q142. Diuretic used in acute hypercalcemia?
Furosemide
After rehydration.

Q143. Aldosterone antagonists effect on acid-base?
Cause acidosis
Reduced H^+ secretion.

Q144. Diuretic safe in nephrotic syndrome with low GFR?
Loop diuretics
Potent enough despite protein binding.

Q145. Renal drug causing gynecomastia and menstrual irregularity?
Spironolactone
Due to antiandrogen effect.

Q146. Drug used to slow CKD in non-diabetic patients (recent trials)?
SGLT2 inhibitors
Eg: dapagliflozin.

Q147. CKD drug that binds phosphate without increasing calcium?
Sevelamer
Non-calcium phosphate binder.

Q148. Thiazide diuretic effect on serum glucose?
May cause hyperglycemia
Due to ↓ insulin secretion.

Q149. Agent used in volume overload and hyponatremia?
Tolvaptan
V2 antagonist.

Q150. Diuretic causing contraction alkalosis?
Loop and thiazide diuretics
Volume loss leads to alkalosis.

Q151. Diuretic causing hyperuricemia and potential gout?
Thiazides
Due to decreased urate excretion.

Q152. Drug causing renal tubular acidosis type 2 (proximal)?
Acetazolamide
Carbonic anhydrase inhibitor → bicarbonate loss.

Q153. Diuretic contraindicated in hepatic encephalopathy?
Acetazolamide
May worsen ammonia retention.

Q154. Nephroprotective effect of RAAS blockers is due to?
Reduction in intraglomerular pressure
Via efferent arteriole dilation.

Q155. Diuretic that increases bicarbonate excretion?
Acetazolamide
Causes metabolic acidosis.

Q156. Electrolyte disturbance with thiazides and loops?
Hypokalemia
Due to increased distal Na^+ delivery.

Q157. Risk when combining ACE inhibitors with K^+-sparing diuretics?
Severe hyperkalemia
Monitor potassium closely.

Q158. IV drug used to manage cerebral edema and high ICP?
Mannitol
Osmotic effect pulls fluid out of brain.

Q159. Antineoplastic agent causing hemorrhagic cystitis?
Ifosfamide
Also managed with MESNA.

Q160. Most common cause of drug-induced acute interstitial nephritis?
NSAIDs and beta-lactams
Allergic-type reaction.

Q161. Renal side effect of amphotericin B?
Renal tubular acidosis + electrolyte wasting
Especially Mg^{2+} and K^+.

Q162. Drug used in SIADH to cause aquaresis?
Tolvaptan
Promotes water loss without sodium loss.

Q163. Key advantage of eplerenone over spironolactone?
Selectivity for aldosterone receptor
Less gynecomastia.

Q164. Drug that inhibits urate reabsorption in proximal tubule?
Probenecid
Uricosuric agent.

Q165. Cause of nephrogenic DI besides lithium?
Demeclocycline
Also used to treat SIADH.

Q166. Diuretic acting on the early distal tubule?
Thiazides
Inhibit Na^+/Cl^- symporter.

Q167. Phosphate binder that can cause iron overload?
Ferric citrate
Dual iron + phosphate-lowering effect.

Q168. Drug that increases risk of uric acid stones?
Loop diuretics
Dehydration and urate concentration.

Q169. Anticoagulant that requires renal dose adjustment?
LMWH (e.g., enoxaparin)
Especially in elderly with low GFR.

Q170. NSAID most nephrotoxic?
Indomethacin
Potent COX inhibitor.

Q171. Antihypertensive that causes reversible renal impairment?
ACE inhibitors
Expected GFR decline <30% is acceptable.

Q172. SGLT2 inhibitors also reduce risk of which renal complication?
Progression to ESRD
Renoprotective effect in multiple trials.

Q173. Antiviral causing Fanconi-like syndrome?
Tenofovir
Proximal tubule toxicity.

Q174. Drug class that may falsely raise creatinine levels?
Trimethoprim and cimetidine
Inhibit tubular creatinine secretion.

Q175. Drug used for metabolic alkalosis in volume overload states?
Acetazolamide
Excretes bicarbonate.

Q176. Bicarbonate is reabsorbed mainly in?
Proximal convoluted tubule
Carbonic anhydrase dependent.

Q177. Diuretic that reduces polyuria in nephrogenic DI?
Thiazides
Paradoxical effect via volume contraction.

Q178. Antidiuretic drug used in central diabetes insipidus?
Desmopressin
V2 agonist.

Q179. Drug that reduces albuminuria in diabetic nephropathy?
ACE inhibitors
Improve outcomes even without HTN.

Q180. SGLT2 inhibitors' unique side effect?
Euglycemic DKA
Rare but serious.

Q181. Key lab marker for monitoring ACEi therapy in CKD?
Serum creatinine and potassium
Monitor after 1–2 weeks.

Q182. SGLT2 inhibitor effect on BP?
Mild antihypertensive
Due to natriuresis and weight loss.

Q183. Drug contraindicated in severe hyponatremia?
Thiazides
May worsen Na^+ loss.

Q184. Diuretic least likely to cause sexual side effects?
Eplerenone
No antiandrogen activity.

Q185. Key side effect of vaptans?
Liver toxicity (esp. tolvaptan)
Monitor LFTs.

Q186. Antihypertensive best suited for renovascular hypertension?
ACE inhibitors
But avoid in bilateral RAS.

Q187. Renal clearance depends on?
Filtration + secretion − reabsorption
Used to calculate drug dosing.

Q188. Hyperkalemia risk drugs (mnemonic)?
K-BANK: K^+-sparing, Beta-blockers, ACEi, NSAIDs, K^+ supplements
High-yield for exams.

Q189. Diuretic safe in allergy to sulfa drugs?
Ethacrynic acid
Non-sulfonamide loop diuretic.

Q190. Diuretic preferred in nephrotic syndrome?
Loop diuretics
Effective even with hypoalbuminemia.

Q191. Diuretic-induced metabolic alkalosis is corrected by?
Acetazolamide
Promotes bicarbonate loss.

Q192. Drug with aquaretic (water only) effect?
Vaptans
Promote free water excretion.

Q193. Drug improving anemia in CKD via HIF stabilization?
Roxadustat
Increases EPO production.

Q194. Most common side effect of phosphate binders?
GI upset
Nausea, bloating, constipation.

Q195. Renal drug combination increasing AKI risk?
ACEi + NSAID + diuretic
Triple whammy.

Q196. Diuretic used in forced alkaline diuresis for poisoning?
Acetazolamide
Enhances bicarbonate excretion.

Q197. Renal marker better than creatinine in early AKI?
Cystatin C
Rises earlier.

Q198. Effect of loop diuretics on calcium?
Increased excretion
May cause hypocalcemia.

Q199. GFR calculation uses which endogenous marker?
Creatinine
Used in MDRD and CKD-EPI formulas.

Q200. Antihypertensive that also reduces albuminuria in CKD?
ARBs
Similar to ACE inhibitors.

Toxicology & Antidotes

Q1. Antidote for acetaminophen overdose?
N-acetylcysteine (NAC)
Replenishes glutathione.

Q2. Antidote for organophosphate poisoning?
Atropine + pralidoxime
Atropine blocks muscarinic effects, pralidoxime reactivates AChE.

Q3. Antidote for benzodiazepine toxicity?
Flumazenil
GABA-A receptor antagonist.

Q4. Antidote for beta-blocker overdose?
Glucagon
Increases cAMP independent of beta-receptors.

Q5. Antidote for calcium channel blocker overdose?
IV calcium + glucagon + high-dose insulin
Supports cardiac function.

Q6. Antidote for digoxin toxicity?
Digoxin-specific antibody fragments (Digibind)
Binds and neutralizes digoxin.

Q7. Antidote for iron overdose?
Deferoxamine
Chelates ferric iron.

Q8. Antidote for methanol or ethylene glycol poisoning?
Fomepizole (or ethanol)
Inhibits alcohol dehydrogenase.

Q9. Antidote for cyanide poisoning?
Hydroxocobalamin
Forms cyanocobalamin (vitamin B12).

Q10. Antidote for heparin overdose?
Protamine sulfate
Positively charged protein.

Q11. Antidote for warfarin overdose?
Vitamin K ± FFP or PCC
Reverses INR.

Q12. Antidote for carbon monoxide poisoning?
100% oxygen or hyperbaric oxygen
Displaces CO from hemoglobin.

Q13. Antidote for opioid overdose?
Naloxone
Rapid reversal of respiratory depression.

Q14. Antidote for isoniazid toxicity?
Pyridoxine (vitamin B6)
Prevents seizures and neurotoxicity.

Q15. Antidote for anticholinergic toxicity (e.g., atropine)?
Physostigmine
Crosses BBB to reverse central effects.

Q16. Antidote for TCA overdose?
Sodium bicarbonate
Reduces cardiotoxicity.

Q17. Antidote for cyanide + CO poisoning (smoke inhalation)?
Hydroxocobalamin
Dual benefit, safe and fast.

Q18. Antidote for arsenic or mercury poisoning?
Dimercaprol (BAL)
Chelates heavy metals.

Q19. Antidote for lead poisoning in children?
Succimer (DMSA)
Oral chelator.

Q20. Treatment for salicylate (aspirin) overdose?
Alkalinization of urine with sodium bicarbonate
Enhances excretion.

Q21. Antidote for fluoride toxicity?
Calcium gluconate
Binds fluoride, prevents hypocalcemia.

Q22. Antidote for methemoglobinemia?
Methylene blue
Converts Fe^{3+} to Fe^{2+} in hemoglobin.

Q23. Antidote for severe copper poisoning (Wilson disease)?
Penicillamine
Chelates copper.

Q24. Toxin that causes cherry red lips and skin?
Carbon monoxide
Binds hemoglobin 200× more than O_2.

Q25. Bitter almond smell suggests poisoning by?
Cyanide
Rapid onset of toxicity.

Q26. Garlic odor in poisoning?
Organophosphates, arsenic
Also found in phosphine gas exposure.

Q27. Rotten egg smell in poisoning?
Hydrogen sulfide
Lethal in high concentration.

Q28. Iron overdose leads to which metabolic disorder?
Anion gap metabolic acidosis
Due to mitochondrial damage.

Q29. Treatment of serotonin syndrome?
Benzodiazepines + cyproheptadine
Supportive care is key.

Q30. Antidote for ethylene glycol toxicity?
Fomepizole
Prevents oxalate formation.

Q31. Chelator contraindicated in iron poisoning?
EDTA
Does not bind iron.

Q32. Signs of TCA overdose?
Wide QRS, anticholinergic effects, seizures
Cardiotoxicity is main concern.

Q33. First-line drug for amphetamine overdose?
Benzodiazepines
Sedation, seizure control.

Q34. Antidote for snake venom bites?
Antivenom
Specific to type/species.

Q35. Antidote for methotrexate toxicity?
Folinic acid (leucovorin)
Rescues normal cells.

Q36. Antidote for sulfonylurea-induced hypoglycemia?
Octreotide
Suppresses insulin release.

Q37. What neutralizes radiation exposure to thyroid?
Potassium iodide (KI)
Blocks uptake of radioactive iodine.

Q38. Early antidote to paracetamol overdose (within 8 hrs)?
N-acetylcysteine
Prevents liver damage.

Q39. Treatment for severe theophylline toxicity?
Activated charcoal + beta-blockers
Control arrhythmias.

Q40. Mechanism of pralidoxime in OP poisoning?
Reactivates acetylcholinesterase
Effective only early.

Q41. Drug causing blue skin and chocolate-colored blood?
Dapsone (methemoglobinemia)
Treat with methylene blue.

Q42. Antidote for dapsone overdose?
Methylene blue + vitamin C
Reverses methemoglobinemia.

Q43. Drug causing garlic breath and Mee's lines?
Arsenic
Also causes sensorimotor neuropathy.

Q44. Toxin causing painful muscle fasciculations and seizures?
Strychnine
Blocks glycine (inhibitory) receptors.

Q45. Common presentation of organophosphate toxicity?
SLUDGE/BBB: Salivation, Lacrimation, Urination, Defecation, GI upset, Emesis / Bronchorrhea, Bradycardia, Bronchospasm.

Q46. Specific reversal agent for dabigatran?
Idarucizumab
Monoclonal antibody fragment.

Q47. Antidote for isopropyl alcohol poisoning?
Supportive only
No specific antidote needed.

Q48. Toxin causing metabolic acidosis + vision loss?
Methanol
Toxic formate metabolites.

Q49. Preferred IV fluid in toxic alcohol poisoning?
Dextrose + bicarbonate
Supportive + correct acidosis.

Q50. Which toxin binds cytochrome oxidase and halts ATP production?
Cyanide
Cellular hypoxia despite normal oxygen.

Q51. Toxin causing garlic odor and QT prolongation?
Arsenic
Causes multisystem failure and neuropathy.

Q52. First-line management of TCA-induced arrhythmia?
IV sodium bicarbonate
Stabilizes cardiac membrane.

Q53. Pupil finding in opioid overdose?
Pinpoint pupils (miosis)
Classic triad: coma, respiratory depression, miosis.

Q54. Antidote for cyanide poisoning when hydroxocobalamin not available?
Sodium nitrite + sodium thiosulfate
Induces methemoglobinemia + detoxifies.

Q55. Substance causing pink-colored skin postmortem?
Carbon monoxide
Carboxyhemoglobin is cherry-pink.

Q56. Lead poisoning in adults classically affects?
Peripheral nerves
Wrist drop, neuropathy, anemia with basophilic stippling.

Q57. First-line chelator for lead poisoning in children?
Succimer
Oral and well-tolerated.

Q58. Clinical clue of cyanosis not improving with oxygen therapy?
Methemoglobinemia
Chocolate-colored blood.

Q59. Most common cause of methemoglobinemia in neonates?
Nitrite-containing foods or water
Risk from contaminated well water.

Q60. Blue-gray skin pigmentation with toxicity of which drug?
Amiodarone
Long-term side effect.

Q61. Aluminum phosphide poisoning causes death due to?
Refractory shock + ARDS
No specific antidote; $MgSO_4$ supportive.

Q62. Most specific test for CO poisoning?
Carboxyhemoglobin level (ABG with co-oximetry)
Pulse oximetry is falsely normal.

Q63. Pupil size in anticholinergic toxicity?
Mydriasis (dilated pupils)
With dry skin, tachycardia, delirium.

Q64. Common herbicide causing lung fibrosis?
Paraquat
No antidote; causes delayed pneumonitis.

Q65. Poison causing bullous skin lesions and hematuria?
Arsenic
Mees' lines, garlic odor, GI distress.

Q66. Poison associated with SLUDGE symptoms?
Organophosphates
Also causes muscle weakness, bradycardia.

Q67. Iron poisoning initial symptoms?
Vomiting, GI bleeding
Followed by latent phase and shock.

Q68. Poison causing rapid heart block and hyperkalemia?
Digitalis (digoxin)
Yellow vision, arrhythmias.

Q69. Poisoning that mimics alcohol but causes severe acidosis?
Methanol or ethylene glycol
Vision loss or renal failure respectively.

Q70. Treatment for isoniazid-induced seizures?
Pyridoxine
IV large dose matched to INH dose.

Q71. Chelator with risk of nephrotoxicity and hypertension?
Deferoxamine
Used in acute iron toxicity.

Q72. Poisoning with the scent of mothballs?
Naphthalene
Causes hemolysis in G6PD-deficient individuals.

Q73. Salicylate poisoning ABG finding?
Mixed respiratory alkalosis + metabolic acidosis
Characteristic biphasic response.

Q74. Antidote that prevents crystalluria in MTX toxicity?
Alkalinization of urine
Along with leucovorin.

Q75. Cocaine toxicity causes which cardiac event?
Myocardial infarction
Via coronary vasospasm.

Q76. Mainstay treatment in organophosphate-induced respiratory failure?
Atropine (high dose)
Titrate to drying of secretions.

Q77. Drug overdose associated with anion gap metabolic acidosis + ketosis, but no hyperglycemia?

Isopropyl alcohol
No lactic or formic acid accumulation.

Q78. Poison causing metabolic acidosis + calcium oxalate crystals?

Ethylene glycol
Renal toxicity hallmark.

Q79. Gas exposure that causes delayed pulmonary edema?

Phosgene
Used in industrial accidents.

Q80. Antidote for TCA-induced seizures?

Benzodiazepines
Safe, effective.

Q81. Toxin causing lead line on gums?

Chronic lead exposure
Burton's line.

Q82. Risk in giving flumazenil for unknown overdose?

Precipitating seizures
Avoid in mixed TCA + BZD overdose.

Q83. Hydrocarbon aspiration management principle?

Supportive care
Avoid emesis/gastric lavage.

Q84. Tricyclic overdose cardiac effect?

QRS prolongation
Risk of arrhythmia.

Q85. Preferred imaging in body packer drug ingestion?

X-ray abdomen
Detects drug packets.

Q86. Drug causing red urine but not hematuria?

Rifampin
Discolors fluids.

Q87. Cherry red skin and seizures suggest?
Cyanide or CO poisoning
Differentiate by setting (e.g., fire exposure).

Q88. First-line treatment for mild salicylate toxicity?
Activated charcoal
If within 1–2 hours.

Q89. Drug that can falsely elevate creatinine in lab tests?
Cefoxitin, trimethoprim
Interferes with assay, not GFR.

Q90. Alcohol withdrawal is treated with?
Benzodiazepines
Preferably long-acting (diazepam).

Q91. Poisoning presenting with garlic breath, GI symptoms, QT prolongation?
Arsenic
Confirm with urine arsenic.

Q92. Drug used to reduce fluoride absorption in toxicity?
Calcium gluconate
Binds fluoride.

Q93. Organophosphate vs carbamate poisoning difference?
Carbamates have shorter duration
Pralidoxime often not needed.

Q94. Organophosphate poisoning test for confirmation?
Plasma pseudocholinesterase level
Decreased in exposure.

Q95. Toxin associated with blue-green vomitus?
Copper sulfate
Also causes GI erosions.

Q96. Substance causing hemorrhagic gastroenteritis + shock?
Iron
Latent phase followed by rapid deterioration.

Q97. Antidote contraindicated in carbamate poisoning?
Pralidoxime (controversial)
Atropine sufficient.

Q98. Antidote for nitrobenzene-induced methemoglobinemia?
Methylene blue
Reduces Fe^{3+} to Fe^{2+}.

Q99. Cocaine overdose with seizures is treated with?
Benzodiazepines
Avoid beta-blockers due to unopposed alpha.

Q100. Bradycardia and hypotension from beta-blocker overdose — treat with?
IV glucagon
Increases intracellular cAMP.

Q101. Bitter almond smell in an unconscious patient indicates?
Cyanide poisoning
Rapid onset, often fatal without antidote.

Q102. Mechanism of cyanide toxicity?
Inhibits cytochrome oxidase (Complex IV)
Halts oxidative phosphorylation → lactic acidosis.

Q103. First-line antidote for cyanide in hospital setting?
Hydroxocobalamin
Converts cyanide to cyanocobalamin.

Q104. Color of blood in CO poisoning?
Bright red
Due to carboxyhemoglobin.

Q105. Visual symptoms with methanol poisoning?
Blurred vision, "snowfield" vision, blindness
Due to formic acid accumulation.

Q106. Metabolic finding in ethylene glycol poisoning?
High anion gap metabolic acidosis
With calcium oxalate crystals.

Q107. GI symptom seen early in iron poisoning?
Vomiting with hematemesis
Corrosive injury to GI mucosa.

Q108. Mechanism of salicylate-induced respiratory alkalosis?
Direct stimulation of respiratory center
Followed by metabolic acidosis.

Q109. Toxicity of dapsone is managed with?
Methylene blue
Treats methemoglobinemia.

Q110. Drug that causes Parkinsonism as a side effect and overdose symptom?
Manganese (in welders)
Extrapyramidal features.

Q111. Which anticonvulsant overdose causes nystagmus and ataxia?
Phenytoin
Common in moderate overdose.

Q112. Toxic alcohol associated with renal failure?
Ethylene glycol
Oxalate crystals cause nephrotoxicity.

Q113. Delayed pulmonary fibrosis after exposure to?
Paraquat
Fatal if not rapidly decontaminated.

Q114. Antidote for lead poisoning with encephalopathy?
Dimercaprol + EDTA
For CNS involvement.

Q115. Chelator for mercury poisoning?
Dimercaprol or succimer
Avoid oral intake with fish/shellfish.

Q116. Poison causing painful tonic seizures and risus sardonicus?
Strychnine
Inhibits glycine at spinal cord.

Q117. Clinical sign of belladonna (atropine) toxicity?
Dry mouth, flushed skin, dilated pupils
"Dry as a bone, red as a beet, blind as a bat…"

Q118. Skin sign in thallium poisoning?
Alopecia
Also painful neuropathy and GI upset.

Q119. Acid-base finding in salicylate poisoning?
Mixed respiratory alkalosis + metabolic acidosis
Classic dual disturbance.

Q120. Common cause of anion gap acidosis with osmolar gap?
Methanol or ethylene glycol
Toxic alcohols.

Q121. Treatment of amphetamine toxicity with agitation?
Benzodiazepines
First-line for CNS and autonomic symptoms.

Q122. Risk of flumazenil in chronic benzodiazepine users?
Seizures
Use with extreme caution.

Q123. Toxin causing bull's-eye maculopathy?
Chloroquine
Irreversible visual loss.

Q124. Early symptom of acute lead toxicity?
Colicky abdominal pain
Often with constipation.

Q125. Most dangerous symptom of TCA overdose?
Arrhythmias
Especially wide QRS complex.

Q126. Drug overdose leading to green vision?
Digoxin
Xanthopsia with arrhythmias.

Q127. Management of massive iron poisoning includes?
Whole bowel irrigation + deferoxamine
GI decontamination is key.

Q128. Effect of salicylate on platelets?
Irreversible inhibition of COX
↑ Bleeding time.

Q129. Tramadol overdose increases risk of?
Seizures
Even in therapeutic doses.

Q130. Drug with toxidrome of sweating, tachycardia, clonus, hyperreflexia?
Serotonin syndrome
From SSRIs, MAOIs, or combinations.

Q131. First-line treatment of serotonin syndrome?
Benzodiazepines
Cyproheptadine if severe.

Q132. Electrolyte imbalance worsening digoxin toxicity?
Hypokalemia
Increases digoxin binding to Na^+/K^+ ATPase.

Q133. Classic toxidrome of opioid overdose?
Pinpoint pupils + respiratory depression + CNS depression
Naloxone is lifesaving.

Q134. Antidote used to reverse NOACs like apixaban?
Andexanet alfa
Decoy Xa protein.

Q135. Drug causing chocolate-colored blood in infants after diarrhea meds?
Dapsone or nitrate exposure
Causes methemoglobinemia.

Q136. Common poison in rural India with high fatality?
Aluminum phosphide
No antidote; causes shock, ARDS.

Q137. Alkali ingestion is more dangerous than acid because?
Causes liquefactive necrosis
Deeper tissue penetration.

Q138. Most common organ damaged by paraquat poisoning?
Lungs
Leads to progressive fibrosis.

Q139. Key finding in nicotine overdose?
Tachycardia → bradycardia, fasciculations
Biphasic effect.

Q140. Antidote for scorpion sting neurotoxicity?
Prazosin
Blocks sympathetic storm.

Q141. Plant alkaloid that inhibits sodium-potassium ATPase?
Digoxin
Narrow therapeutic window.

Q142. Drug that may cause cyanide poisoning on overdose?
Nitroprusside
Especially with prolonged high-dose infusion.

Q143. Antidote for nitroprusside-induced cyanide toxicity?
Hydroxocobalamin
Or sodium thiosulfate.

Q144. Clinical use of milk in poisoning?
Soothing for mild corrosive intake
Not an antidote.

Q145. Eye finding in methanol toxicity?
Retinal hyperemia
Followed by optic atrophy.

Q146. Treatment for arsenic-induced peripheral neuropathy?
Dimercaprol or succimer
Early chelation helps.

Q147. Management of hydrocarbon ingestion?
Supportive only
Aspiration risk; avoid lavage.

Q148. Lactic acidosis in well-oxygenated patient suggests?
Cyanide poisoning
No cellular respiration.

Q149. Treatment of phenobarbital overdose?
Urine alkalinization
Enhances excretion.

Q150. Antidote for ethylene glycol toxicity?
Fomepizole
Prevents oxalate metabolite formation.

Q151. What is the antidote for digoxin-induced arrhythmias?
Digoxin-specific antibody fragments (Digibind)
Binds free digoxin and neutralizes it.

Q152. Poison causing lactic acidosis with normal oxygen saturation?
Cyanide
Cellular hypoxia despite normal SpO_2.

Q153. Toxicity presenting with gum lines, anemia, and wrist drop?
Lead
Also causes basophilic stippling.

Q154. Specific sign of carbon monoxide poisoning?
Cherry-red lips and mucosa
But often not seen clinically.

Q155. Which poison causes garlic breath and Mee's lines on nails?
Arsenic
Also neuropathy and QT prolongation.

Q156. First-line therapy in isoniazid-induced seizures?
Pyridoxine (Vitamin B6)
Equal to the ingested dose of INH.

Q157. Characteristic breath odor in ethanol poisoning?
Fruity or alcoholic
May mask other poisonings.

Q158. Common herbicide causing lung fibrosis and multiorgan failure?
Paraquat
Very lethal; avoid oxygen unless necessary.

Q159. CNS stimulant overdose treated with which class of drugs?
Benzodiazepines
Controls agitation, seizures, BP.

Q160. Brown blood not responding to oxygen therapy suggests?
Methemoglobinemia
Treat with methylene blue.

Q161. Toxin causing renal stones and hypocalcemia?
Ethylene glycol
Calcium oxalate crystals in urine.

Q162. Pesticide exposure causing muscarinic symptoms and miosis?
Organophosphates
Treat with atropine + pralidoxime.

Q163. Which gas is known as "silent killer"?
Carbon monoxide
Colorless, odorless, binds Hb.

Q164. Toxin causing bradycardia, hypotension, and AV block?
Beta-blockers
Treat with glucagon.

Q165. Common side effect of naloxone administration?
Withdrawal symptoms
Restlessness, vomiting, hypertension.

Q166. Cyanide poisoning antidote that works by forming methemoglobin?
Sodium nitrite
Converts hemoglobin to methemoglobin.

Q167. Drug overdose causing horizontal nystagmus and ataxia?
Phenytoin
Toxicity includes cerebellar signs.

Q168. Most common cause of acute liver failure in adults?
Acetaminophen overdose
NAC is lifesaving.

Q169. Hemodialysis is most useful in which poisoning?
Methanol, ethylene glycol, lithium
Low molecular weight, water-soluble toxins.

Q170. Sign of corrosive acid ingestion?
Oral burns, drooling, stridor
Avoid inducing vomiting.

Q171. Drug causing bradycardia with blue skin discoloration on overdose?
Amiodarone
Chronic use side effect.

Q172. Poisoning with tremor, tachycardia, fever, and hyperreflexia?
Serotonin syndrome
Treat with benzodiazepines ± cyproheptadine.

Q173. Overdose of which drug is treated with leucovorin rescue?
Methotrexate
Folinic acid bypasses DHFR blockade.

Q174. First sign of atropine overdose?
Dry mouth
Anticholinergic toxidrome.

Q175. Rat poison containing superwarfarin is reversed by?
High-dose vitamin K + FFP
May need prolonged therapy.

Q176. Sign of acute salicylate poisoning in children?
Tinnitus, vomiting, hyperventilation
Mixed acid-base disturbance.

Q177. First-line in hydrocarbon ingestion with no vomiting?
Observation
Avoid lavage or emetics.

Q178. Which heavy metal inhibits sulfhydryl enzymes and causes neuropathy?
Lead
Especially in industrial exposure.

Q179. Antidote for fluoride ingestion (toothpaste overdose)?
Calcium gluconate
Binds free fluoride.

Q180. Highly protein-bound drug causing arrhythmia and visual changes?
Digoxin
Treat with Digibind.

Q181. Classical skin lesion of arsenic toxicity?
Hyperkeratosis of palms/soles
Seen in chronic exposure.

Q182. Immediate priority in cyanide poisoning?
100% oxygen
Followed by antidote administration.

Q183. Urinary finding in ethylene glycol poisoning?
Calcium oxalate crystals
Envelope or needle-shaped.

Q184. Sodium channel blocker effect on ECG?
Widened QRS
Seen in TCA overdose.

Q185. Primary effect of organophosphates on autonomic system?
Parasympathetic overactivity
SLUDGE symptoms.

Q186. Hallmark symptom of serotonin syndrome but not in NMS?
Clonus
NMS has lead-pipe rigidity.

Q187. Drug that may cause cyanide toxicity with prolonged use?
Nitroprusside
More in renal failure.

Q188. First aid for corrosive alkali ingestion?
Do not induce vomiting; give milk
Endoscopy after stabilization.

Q189. Classic cardiac marker for cocaine toxicity?
ST elevation, MI
Due to vasospasm.

Q190. Overdose presenting with anion gap acidosis and ketones, no glucose elevation?
Isopropyl alcohol
Managed supportively.

Q191. Drug causing miosis, bradycardia, and drowsiness in overdose?
Opioids
Respiratory depression follows.

Q192. CNS effect of aluminum phosphide poisoning?
Delirium, coma
Alongside circulatory collapse.

Q193. Toxin causing "pink tooth" postmortem?
Carbon monoxide
Rare but classical finding.

Q194. Activated charcoal is ineffective in which poisoning?
Iron, lithium, alcohol
Not bound by charcoal.

Q195. First-line for phenobarbital overdose?
Urinary alkalinization
Increases excretion.

Q196. Clinical clue for cyanide poisoning in smoke inhalation?

Rapid onset coma, lactic acidosis

Especially in enclosed space fires.

Q197. Drug overdose with ECG: bradycardia + hyperkalemia + scooped ST?

Digoxin

"Salvador Dali's moustache" ST depression.

Q198. Most common cause of drug-induced methemoglobinemia?

Dapsone

Treated with methylene blue.

Q199. What increases risk of acetaminophen toxicity in alcoholics?

Glutathione depletion

Chronic alcohol use lowers reserves.

Q200. Safe and effective way to enhance excretion of weak acids (e.g. phenobarbital)?

Alkalinization of urine

Enhances ion trapping.

Autacoids & Anti-inflammatory Drugs

Q1. Main receptor involved in gastric acid secretion by histamine?
H2 receptor
Stimulates parietal cells in the stomach.

Q2. Drug used to prevent NSAID-induced ulcers?
Misoprostol
Prostaglandin E1 analog.

Q3. Which prostaglandin causes uterine contraction?
$PGF_2\alpha$
Used in obstetrics to induce labor.

Q4. Aspirin irreversibly inhibits which enzyme?
Cyclooxygenase (COX-1 and COX-2)
Inhibits thromboxane A2 synthesis.

Q5. Selective COX-2 inhibitor with less GI side effects?
Celecoxib
Increased risk of thrombosis.

Q6. Which leukotriene causes bronchoconstriction?
LTC_4, LTD_4
Potent mediators in asthma.

Q7. Drug used to prevent aspirin-induced asthma?
Montelukast
Leukotriene receptor antagonist.

Q8. Drug used to close PDA in neonates?
Indomethacin
Inhibits PGE_2 synthesis.

Q9. Drug used to keep PDA open in congenital heart defects?
Alprostadil (PGE_1)
Maintains ductal patency.

Q10. Antipyretic and analgesic that lacks anti-inflammatory effect?
Paracetamol
Acts centrally, minimal COX inhibition peripherally.

Q11. Antidote for paracetamol overdose?
N-acetylcysteine
Replenishes glutathione.

Q12. Drug that blocks 5-HT_3 receptors to treat chemotherapy-induced vomiting?
Ondansetron
Centrally acting antiemetic.

Q13. 5-HT_1 agonist used for migraine treatment?
Sumatriptan
Causes vasoconstriction of cerebral vessels.

Q14. Which NSAID is safest in pregnancy?
Paracetamol
NSAIDs should be avoided especially in 3rd trimester.

Q15. Long-term NSAID use may cause what renal complication?
Papillary necrosis
Due to reduced prostaglandins.

Q16. Which NSAID is highly nephrotoxic and avoided in CKD?
Indomethacin
Potent COX inhibitor.

Q17. Which antihistamine causes maximum sedation?
Diphenhydramine
First-generation H1 blocker.

Q18. Second-generation antihistamine with minimal sedation?
Loratadine
Does not cross BBB.

Q19. Which prostaglandin is used to induce abortion?
Misoprostol
Causes uterine contractions.

Q20. 5-HT_2 antagonist used in carcinoid syndrome?
Cyproheptadine
Also used for serotonin syndrome.

Q21. Bradykinin antagonist used in hereditary angioedema?
Icatibant
B2 receptor antagonist.

Q22. Why is aspirin contraindicated in children with viral fever?
Reye's syndrome
Hepatic failure + encephalopathy.

Q23. Which NSAID inhibits both COX and lipoxygenase?
Licofelone (under trial)
Experimental dual inhibitor.

Q24. Most potent NSAID for acute gout attack?
Indomethacin
Also reduces inflammation.

Q25. NSAID that does not affect platelet function?
Celecoxib
No COX-1 inhibition.

Q26. Main prostaglandin involved in fever?
PGE_2
Acts on hypothalamus.

Q27. Drug used to delay preterm labor?
Tocolytics like nifedipine; previously used indomethacin
Indomethacin inhibits PGs.

Q28. Common GI side effect of NSAIDs?
Gastric ulcers
Due to COX-1 inhibition.

Q29. Mechanism of antipyresis by paracetamol?
Inhibits hypothalamic prostaglandin synthesis
Centrally acting.

Q30. Which serotonin receptor is a target for anti-migraine therapy?
$5\text{-}HT_1B/1D$
Triptans act here.

Q31. H1 antihistamines used in motion sickness?
Promethazine, dimenhydrinate
Anticholinergic action.

Q32. Which NSAID is contraindicated in aspirin-sensitive asthma?
All non-selective NSAIDs
May cause bronchospasm.

Q33. Long-acting leukotriene receptor antagonist?
Montelukast
Taken once daily.

Q34. 5-HT_3 antagonist used in IBS-D?
Alosetron
Risk of ischemic colitis.

Q35. NSAID with lowest cardiovascular risk?
Naproxen
COX-1 preference reduces CV risk.

Q36. Most common side effect of H2 blockers?
Diarrhea, headache
Gynecomastia (cimetidine) is rare but notable.

Q37. H2 blocker with anti-androgenic effect?
Cimetidine
Causes gynecomastia, ↓ libido.

Q38. Which prostaglandin causes vasodilation and inhibits platelet aggregation?
PGI_2 (prostacyclin)
Opposes TXA_2.

Q39. Antihistamine safe in elderly with BPH?
Loratadine
Minimal anticholinergic action.

Q40. Role of leukotrienes in asthma?
Bronchoconstriction, mucus production
Potent pro-inflammatory mediators.

Q41. Anti-leukotriene drug used in aspirin-sensitive asthma?
Montelukast
Blocks LTD_4 receptors.

Q42. Most common side effect of montelukast?
Headache
Rarely causes neuropsychiatric symptoms.

Q43. Drug used in systemic mastocytosis?
H1 and H2 blockers
Reduce histamine-related symptoms.

Q44. NSAID that is prodrug and less GI irritating?
Nabumetone
COX-2 selective after activation.

Q45. PG analog used for erectile dysfunction?
Alprostadil (PGE_1)
Intracavernosal injection.

Q46. Drug causing tinnitus on overdose?
Aspirin (salicylates)
Early sign of toxicity.

Q47. Use of misoprostol in obstetrics?
Induction of labor, abortion
Uterotonic via PG receptor.

Q48. Prostaglandin used in pulmonary hypertension?
Epoprostenol
PGI_2 analog – vasodilator.

Q49. NSAID contraindicated in CABG patients?
Celecoxib
Risk of thrombosis.

Q50. Role of histamine H3 receptor?
Presynaptic inhibition of histamine release
Modulates neurotransmission.

Q51. NSAID with high risk of hepatotoxicity in overdose?
Paracetamol
Dose-dependent liver necrosis.

Q52. Which drug blocks TXA_2 formation without affecting PGI_2?
Low-dose aspirin
Selectively inhibits COX-1 in platelets.

Q53. Antihistamine that prolongs QT interval?
Terfenadine (withdrawn)
Risk of torsades de pointes.

Q54. H1 blocker with longest duration of action?
Fexofenadine
Once daily dosing.

Q55. Drug useful in urticaria with daytime activity?
Loratadine
Non-sedating.

Q56. Leukotriene pathway inhibitor used in asthma prophylaxis?
Zileuton
5-lipoxygenase inhibitor.

Q57. Use of aspirin in low doses is due to its effect on?
Thromboxane A2
Antiplatelet action.

Q58. PG analog used for glaucoma?
Latanoprost
Increases uveoscleral outflow.

Q59. Side effect of latanoprost?
Iris pigmentation
Brown discoloration.

Q60. Major side effect of cimetidine in males?
Gynecomastia
Anti-androgenic.

Q61. H1 blockers with maximum anticholinergic effect?
Promethazine
Also used in motion sickness.

Q62. Aspirin triad includes asthma, nasal polyps, and?
Aspirin sensitivity
Seen in some atopic individuals.

Q63. Bradykinin accumulation occurs with which drug?
ACE inhibitors
Causes dry cough and angioedema.

Q64. Which eicosanoid causes platelet aggregation?
Thromboxane A2
Formed by COX-1.

Q65. Prostaglandin used to ripen cervix before delivery?
Dinoprostone (PGE_2)
Softens cervix.

Q66. Which NSAID is highly protein bound and interacts with warfarin?
Diclofenac
Displaces protein-bound drugs.

Q67. Mechanism of action of montelukast?
Blocks leukotriene D_4 receptor
Reduces bronchoconstriction.

Q68. Main role of PGI_2 in vasculature?
Vasodilation, anti-platelet
Opposes thromboxane.

Q69. In asthma, leukotrienes are produced by?
Mast cells, eosinophils
LTC_4, LTD_4, LTE_4 involved.

Q70. Common cause of urticaria after taking NSAIDs?
Non-immunologic mast cell degranulation
COX inhibition shifts AA pathway.

Q71. First-generation H1 blockers cross BBB because?
Lipophilic nature
Cause drowsiness.

Q72. NSAID safe in bleeding disorder?
Paracetamol
No antiplatelet action.

Q73. Common prostaglandin used to treat postpartum hemorrhage?
Carboprost
$PGF2\alpha$ analog.

Q74. Which PG analog is used to prevent NSAID-induced gastric ulcers?
Misoprostol
Also causes diarrhea.

Q75. Why are selective COX-2 inhibitors not fully safe?
No TXA2 inhibition → thrombosis
Imbalance between PGI2 and TXA2.

Q76. Drug used in cluster headaches targeting 5-HT1B/1D?
Sumatriptan
Constricts cranial vessels.

Q77. NSAID with very short half-life but strong analgesia?
Ketorolac
Used for post-op pain.

Q78. Antihistamine that also treats anxiety and insomnia?
Hydroxyzine
Sedating antihistamine.

Q79. Histamine receptor responsible for motion sickness?
H1
In vestibular system.

Q80. Common GI side effect of COX inhibitors?
Gastritis, ulcer
COX-1 protects mucosa.

Q81. Which PG analog is used in erectile dysfunction?
Alprostadil
PGE1 analog.

Q82. Drug for NSAID-induced renal injury prevention?
Misoprostol (theoretically), or avoiding NSAIDs
PGs maintain renal perfusion.

Q83. Misoprostol-induced diarrhea is due to?
PGE_1 effect on GI smooth muscle
Increases motility.

Q84. Which leukotriene receptor antagonist has hepatic toxicity risk?
Zileuton
Requires LFT monitoring.

Q85. PGI_2 analog used in pulmonary hypertension?
Epoprostenol
Vasodilator + platelet inhibitor.

Q86. NSAID with longest half-life?
Piroxicam
Once-daily dosing.

Q87. Which PG analog used to maintain PDA?
Alprostadil
Keeps ductus arteriosus open.

Q88. COX isoform induced by inflammation?
COX-2
COX-1 is constitutive.

Q89. Drug used in aspirin-induced asthma prophylaxis?
Montelukast
Prevents leukotriene-mediated bronchospasm.

Q90. PG analog used for glaucoma with once-daily dosing?
Latanoprost
Reduces intraocular pressure.

Q91. Histamine receptor causing gastric acid secretion?
H2
Targeted by ranitidine, famotidine.

Q92. Drug that causes cross-sensitivity with aspirin in asthma?
All non-selective NSAIDs
Celecoxib is safer.

Q93. Role of thromboxane in clotting?
Platelet aggregation and vasoconstriction
From COX-1 in platelets.

Q94. Antipyretic action of NSAIDs is due to inhibition of?
PGE_2 synthesis in hypothalamus
Resetting the thermostat.

Q95. Use of cyproheptadine in serotonin syndrome?
$5\text{-}HT_2$ antagonist
Reverses serotonin excess.

Q96. First-line treatment for NSAID-induced gastritis?
PPIs (e.g., omeprazole)
More effective than H2 blockers.

Q97. NSAID with maximum risk of GI bleed?

Ketorolac

Avoid long-term use.

Q98. Leukotriene receptor antagonists block which leukotrienes?

LTD_4, LTE_4

Via $CysLT_1$ receptor.

Q99. Drug used in hereditary angioedema targeting bradykinin?

Icatibant

B_2 receptor blocker.

Q100. Which serotonin receptor causes vasoconstriction?

$5\text{-}HT_1B$

Target of triptans.

Q101. Which prostaglandin causes diarrhea as a side effect?

Misoprostol

Stimulates GI smooth muscle.

Q102. Antihistamine used in anaphylaxis?

Diphenhydramine (IV)

Given after epinephrine.

Q103. Mechanism of epinephrine in anaphylaxis?

$\beta 2$ bronchodilation + α vasoconstriction

Rapid reversal of airway collapse.

Q104. H1 blocker with maximum anticholinergic activity?

Promethazine

Causes dry mouth, sedation.

Q105. NSAID that causes minimal GI side effects?

Celecoxib

COX-2 selective.

Q106. Drug causing irreversible COX inhibition?

Aspirin

Only NSAID with this property.

Q107. NSAID safe for short-term use in post-op pain?

Ketorolac

Avoid >5 days due to GI/renal toxicity.

Q108. Leukotriene antagonist useful in allergic rhinitis?
Montelukast
Also used in asthma prophylaxis.

Q109. PG analog causing uterine contractions + abortion?
Misoprostol
Used with mifepristone.

Q110. Drug used for labor induction and cervical ripening?
Dinoprostone
PGE_2 analog.

Q111. Role of LTC_4 in asthma?
Bronchoconstriction + ↑ mucus
Targeted by montelukast.

Q112. 5-HT_3 antagonist used as antiemetic?
Ondansetron
Acts on CTZ and GI tract.

Q113. Leukotriene pathway enzyme inhibited by zileuton?
5-lipoxygenase
Reduces all leukotriene synthesis.

Q114. PG analog used in male erectile dysfunction?
Alprostadil
PGE_1 causes vasodilation.

Q115. PG analog used in glaucoma that increases outflow?
Latanoprost
PGF2α analog.

Q116. H1 blockers effective in motion sickness due to?
Anticholinergic property
Vestibular pathway involvement.

Q117. Which PG causes fever by acting on hypothalamus?
PGE_2
Central pyrogenic mediator.

Q118. Commonest cause of drug-induced urticaria?
NSAIDs
Especially non-selective ones.

Q119. COX-2 selective NSAID with lowest GI risk?
Etoricoxib
Similar efficacy to celecoxib.

Q120. Drug that inhibits platelet aggregation but not inflammation?
Low-dose aspirin
Irreversible TXA2 inhibition.

Q121. Antihistamine with antiserotonin property?
Cyproheptadine
Used in carcinoid syndrome, appetite stimulant.

Q122. NSAID safe in hemophilia?
Paracetamol
Avoid aspirin and other NSAIDs.

Q123. PG analog contraindicated in pregnancy due to abortion risk?
Misoprostol
Uterine stimulant.

Q124. NSAID with high CV risk profile?
Rofecoxib (withdrawn)
COX-2 only → unopposed thromboxane.

Q125. Anti-inflammatory effect of NSAIDs is due to inhibition of?
Prostaglandins
Especially PGE_2.

Q126. NSAID with maximum enterohepatic circulation?
Piroxicam
Long half-life, once daily.

Q127. Use of montelukast in exercise-induced asthma?
Prevents bronchospasm
Taken 2 hours before activity.

Q128. Use of sumatriptan is contraindicated in?
Ischemic heart disease
Coronary vasospasm risk.

Q129. PG analog used to delay preterm labor?
Indomethacin (NSAID)
Inhibits prostaglandins.

Q130. Drug causing tinnitus and respiratory alkalosis in overdose?
Aspirin
Early salicylate poisoning.

Q131. Antihistamine with mast cell-stabilizing effect?
Ketotifen
Prevents histamine release.

Q132. PG analog given intraurethrally for ED?
Alprostadil
Acts via cAMP.

Q133. PGE_1 analog used for cervical priming?
Misoprostol
Also used for postpartum hemorrhage.

Q134. Use of PGF2α analog in obstetrics?
Carboprost
Uterine contractions + control bleeding.

Q135. Which eicosanoid is bronchoprotective?
PGI_2
Vasodilator and platelet inhibitor.

Q136. Preferred NSAID in gout with CV risk?
Naproxen
Least CV side effects.

Q137. Receptor target of loratadine?
H1 receptor
Minimal CNS penetration.

Q138. Histamine action via H1 receptor includes?
Vasodilation, itching, bronchospasm
Classic allergy mediator.

Q139. Why is aspirin avoided in dengue?
Platelet dysfunction + bleeding risk
Use paracetamol instead.

Q140. Epoprostenol is administered via?
IV infusion
Short half-life requires continuous dosing.

Q141. Risk of abrupt paracetamol withdrawal in chronic users?
Rare withdrawal headache
Not addictive.

Q142. Which drug reduces inflammation without affecting fever or pain?
Glucocorticoids
Strong anti-inflammatory.

Q143. Montelukast acts on which receptor?
$CysLT_1$
Leukotriene D_4 receptor.

Q144. PG analog used in Raynaud's and digital ulcers?
Iloprost
Vasodilator.

Q145. NSAID that causes aseptic meningitis?
Ibuprofen
Rare hypersensitivity.

Q146. H1 blocker with strong sedative and antiemetic action?
Promethazine
Also used in vertigo.

Q147. Bradykinin-mediated angioedema treated by?
Icatibant
B2 antagonist.

Q148. Leukotriene antagonist used in pediatric asthma?
Montelukast
Safe in children >6 months.

Q149. Drug with dual COX and LOX inhibition (experimental)?
Licofelone
Reduces inflammation more completely.

Q150. Action of prostacyclin (PGI_2) in platelets?
Inhibits aggregation
Vasodilator and antithrombotic.

Q151. Which drug inhibits histamine release from mast cells?
Cromolyn sodium
Stabilizes mast cell membranes.

Q152. PG analog used for neonatal ductus arteriosus patency?
Alprostadil
Maintains PDA in congenital heart defects.

Q153. Drug used to reverse NSAID-induced gastric injury?
Misoprostol
Replaces lost PGE_1.

Q154. H1 blocker used in insomnia management?
Diphenhydramine
OTC sleep aid due to sedative effect.

Q155. Drug-induced bronchospasm via COX inhibition suggests?
Aspirin-sensitive asthma
Shift to leukotriene pathway.

Q156. NSAID useful in familial adenomatous polyposis (FAP)?
Celecoxib
Reduces polyp burden.

Q157. Montelukast is contraindicated in which psychiatric condition?
Severe depression/suicidality
Rare neuropsychiatric effects.

Q158. PG analog used to treat impotence?
Alprostadil
Increases cAMP → vasodilation.

Q159. NSAID with high hepatotoxicity risk if overdosed?
Paracetamol
Risk above 150 mg/kg.

Q160. H1 antihistamine least likely to cause sedation?
Fexofenadine
Poor CNS penetration.

Q161. PG analog contraindicated in pregnancy due to uterine contraction?
Misoprostol
Risk of abortion.

Q162. Mechanism of anti-pyresis by NSAIDs?
Inhibition of hypothalamic PGE_2
Resets temperature set point.

Q163. Which PG promotes platelet aggregation and vasoconstriction?
TXA_2
COX-1 product in platelets.

Q164. Which PG opposes thromboxane and prevents clotting?
PGI_2 (prostacyclin)
From vascular endothelium.

Q165. 5-HT_1D receptor agonist used in migraine?
Sumatriptan
Constricts cerebral vessels.

Q166. Drug used to manage carcinoid tumor diarrhea?
Cyproheptadine
Blocks serotonin receptors.

Q167. PG analog that promotes gastric mucus and bicarbonate?
Misoprostol
Cytoprotective.

Q168. Antihistamine with anti-motion sickness effect and sedation?
Dimenhydrinate
First-gen H1 blocker.

Q169. PG analog used in open-angle glaucoma?
Latanoprost
PGF2α analog.

Q170. Which eicosanoid contributes to inflammation and bronchoconstriction?
Leukotriene D_4
Mediator in asthma.

Q171. PGE_2 analog used in cervical dilation?
Dinoprostone
For labor induction.

Q172. NSAID causing least renal damage?
Naproxen (relative)
All NSAIDs risky in CKD.

Q173. Antihistamine with least CNS penetration?
Desloratadine
Long-acting, nonsedating.

Q174. NSAID causing maximum GI ulceration?
Indomethacin
Potent COX inhibitor.

Q175. PGI_2 analog for severe PAH (pulmonary arterial hypertension)?
Epoprostenol
Improves exercise tolerance.

Q176. Cimetidine can inhibit metabolism of which drugs?
Warfarin, phenytoin, theophylline
CYP450 inhibitor.

Q177. Common CNS effect of first-gen antihistamines?
Drowsiness
Used as OTC sleep aid.

Q178. Drug of choice for acute migraine?
Sumatriptan
Fast-acting 5-HT_1 agonist.

Q179. Prostaglandin associated with uterine pain during menses?
PGF2α
Causes dysmenorrhea.

Q180. Drug used to treat NSAID-induced gastritis during pregnancy?
Omeprazole
Safer than misoprostol.

Q181. Antihistamine with appetite stimulant property?
Cyproheptadine
Blocks 5-HT_2 and H1.

Q182. NSAID used topically in ophthalmic inflammation?
Ketorolac
Used post-cataract surgery.

Q183. Drug contraindicated in glaucoma due to mydriasis?
First-gen H1 blockers
Anticholinergic effect.

Q184. NSAID safe in breastfeeding mothers?
Ibuprofen
Minimal secretion in breast milk.

Q185. PGI_2 analog that improves symptoms in systemic sclerosis?
Iloprost
Improves Raynaud's.

Q186. Action of Zileuton in asthma?
Inhibits 5-lipoxygenase
Prevents leukotriene synthesis.

Q187. Best treatment for motion sickness in pregnancy?
Doxylamine + pyridoxine
Safe first-line.

Q188. Serotonin syndrome presents with?
Clonus, hyperreflexia, agitation
Treat with cyproheptadine.

Q189. Anti-inflammatory use of aspirin is dose-dependent. What dose is needed?
>3 g/day
Lower doses for antiplatelet effect.

Q190. Paracetamol is preferred in peptic ulcer because?
No COX-1 inhibition
Minimal GI risk.

Q191. Most potent vasoconstrictive PG?
TXA_2
Stimulates platelet aggregation.

Q192. PG used in renal transplant to maintain renal blood flow?
PGE_1
Vasodilation improves perfusion.

Q193. PG that enhances uterine tone in obstetrics?
$PGF2\alpha$
Carboprost used in PPH.

Q194. Drug for urticaria with minimal sedation?
Fexofenadine
Preferred in working adults.

Q195. First-line drug for primary dysmenorrhea?
NSAIDs (mefenamic acid, ibuprofen)
Block PGF2α.

Q196. Which antihistamine causes paradoxical stimulation in children?
Diphenhydramine
Rare CNS excitatory reaction.

Q197. PG analog used in Buerger disease for ischemia?
Iloprost
Improves microcirculation.

Q198. Drug with both anti-serotonin and anti-histamine effect?
Cyproheptadine
Useful in serotonin syndrome and allergy.

Q199. Antihistamine most effective for rhinitis with sleep disturbance?
Diphenhydramine
Sedating and anti-allergic.

Q200. Which NSAID is preferred in juvenile arthritis?
Naproxen
Approved for pediatric use.

Miscellaneous Pharmacology

Q1. Drug of choice for heavy metal poisoning in Wilson disease?
Penicillamine
Chelates copper.

Q2. Antidote for methotrexate toxicity?
Leucovorin (folinic acid)
Bypasses dihydrofolate reductase.

Q3. Antidote for cyanide poisoning?
Hydroxocobalamin
Converts cyanide to cyanocobalamin.

Q4. Antidote for ethylene glycol poisoning?
Fomepizole
Inhibits alcohol dehydrogenase.

Q5. Antidote for organophosphate poisoning?
Atropine + pralidoxime
Atropine for symptoms; pralidoxime for AChE reactivation.

Q6. Which agent is used for chelation of iron overload?
Deferoxamine
Also used in iron poisoning.

Q7. Which immunosuppressant inhibits IL-2 production?
Cyclosporine
Calcineurin inhibitor.

Q8. Which immunosuppressant causes gum hypertrophy?
Cyclosporine
Also nephrotoxic.

Q9. Which drug is an mTOR inhibitor used in transplantation?
Sirolimus
Inhibits T-cell proliferation.

Q10. Which cytokine is inhibited by tocilizumab?
IL-6
Used in rheumatoid arthritis, cytokine storm.

Q11. Antiretroviral causing nephrolithiasis?
Indinavir
A protease inhibitor.

Q12. Drug used for estrogen receptor-positive breast cancer?
Tamoxifen
SERM.

Q13. Drug used for HER2-positive breast cancer?
Trastuzumab
Monoclonal antibody.

Q14. Monoclonal antibody targeting VEGF?
Bevacizumab
Anti-angiogenic.

Q15. Which drug inhibits xanthine oxidase?
Allopurinol
Used in gout.

Q16. Drug used in tumor lysis syndrome to reduce uric acid rapidly?
Rasburicase
Converts uric acid to allantoin.

Q17. Drug of choice in scorpion sting neurotoxicity in India?
Prazosin
Alpha-blocker.

Q18. Drug used to reduce postpartum hemorrhage via oxytocin receptor?
Oxytocin
Causes uterine contraction.

Q19. Treatment for hyperammonemia in urea cycle disorders?
Sodium benzoate
Converts ammonia to excretable compound.

Q20. Drug for neurocysticercosis?
Albendazole + steroids
Controls parasite + inflammation.

Q21. Drug used in PPH that is contraindicated in asthma?
Carboprost (PGF2α)
Causes bronchospasm.

Q22. Which vitamin deficiency occurs with isoniazid?
Pyridoxine (B6)
Causes peripheral neuropathy.

Q23. Commonest drug to cause gynecomastia?
Spironolactone
Also cimetidine, ketoconazole.

Q24. Drug used in acromegaly treatment?
Octreotide
Somatostatin analog.

Q25. Drug that can cause blue discoloration of vision?
Sildenafil
PDE5 inhibitor.

Q26. Use of dantrolene?
Malignant hyperthermia
Reduces calcium release.

Q27. Antidote for heparin overdose?
Protamine sulfate
Binds heparin.

Q28. Antidote for warfarin overdose?
Vitamin K + FFP/PCC
Restores clotting.

Q29. Drug used to treat serotonin syndrome?
Cyproheptadine
5-HT_2 antagonist.

Q30. Drug causing serotonin syndrome when combined with MAO inhibitors?
Linezolid
Weak MAO inhibitor.

Q31. Drug used for pheochromocytoma pre-op prep?
Phenoxybenzamine
Irreversible α-blocker.

Q32. Anticoagulant safe in pregnancy?
Heparin
Does not cross placenta.

Q33. Antiplatelet agent causing irreversible platelet inhibition?
Aspirin
Inhibits COX-1.

Q34. Drug causing ototoxicity and nephrotoxicity?
Aminoglycosides
Especially with loop diuretics.

Q35. Monoclonal antibody used in psoriasis targeting IL-17?
Secukinumab
For severe plaque psoriasis.

Q36. Drug causing Stevens-Johnson syndrome as adverse effect?
Lamotrigine
Also sulfa drugs, phenytoin.

Q37. Antidiabetic drug with cardioprotective benefit?
Empagliflozin
SGLT2 inhibitor.

Q38. Oral hypoglycemic causing lactic acidosis?
Metformin
Risk ↑ in renal impairment.

Q39. Drug used to promote bone growth in osteoporosis?
Teriparatide
PTH analog.

Q40. Drug of choice for pituitary prolactinoma?
Cabergoline
Dopamine agonist.

Q41. Which drug causes agranulocytosis as side effect?
Clozapine
Also methimazole, carbimazole.

Q42. Drug class causing lupus-like syndrome?
Hydralazine, procainamide
Also INH.

Q43. Biologic used in rheumatoid arthritis targeting TNF-α?
Etanercept
Fusion protein.

Q44. Drug causing pulmonary fibrosis?
Amiodarone, bleomycin
Also methotrexate.

Q45. Drug used for sickle cell anemia to ↑ HbF?
Hydroxyurea
Prevents crises.

Q46. Drug causing grey baby syndrome?
Chloramphenicol
Due to UDP-glucuronyl transferase deficiency.

Q47. Antiretroviral with bone marrow suppression?
Zidovudine
Causes anemia, neutropenia.

Q48. Drug that prolongs QT and used in malaria?
Chloroquine
Monitor ECG.

Q49. Drug of choice for methemoglobinemia?
Methylene blue
Reduces Fe^{3+} to Fe^{2+}.

Q50. Drug used to prevent chemotherapy-induced neutropenia?
Filgrastim (G-CSF)
Stimulates neutrophil recovery.

Q51. Drug used to treat SIADH (Syndrome of Inappropriate ADH)?
Tolvaptan
V2 receptor antagonist.

Q52. Best drug for motion sickness in pregnancy?
Doxylamine + pyridoxine
Safe category A.

Q53. Drug causing gingival hyperplasia and hirsutism?
Phenytoin
Chronic use effect.

Q54. Vitamin used to reduce isoniazid-induced neuropathy?
Pyridoxine (Vitamin B6)
Always co-prescribed.

Q55. Drug used to diagnose myasthenia gravis?
Edrophonium
Short-acting AChE inhibitor.

Q56. Drug used to treat myasthenia gravis long-term?
Pyridostigmine
Does not cross BBB.

Q57. Antidote for benzodiazepine toxicity?
Flumazenil
Competitive GABA-A antagonist.

Q58. Antidote for beta-blocker overdose?
Glucagon
Increases cAMP via non-adrenergic path.

Q59. Drug used to reverse NM blockade by non-depolarizing agents?
Neostigmine
AChE inhibitor.

Q60. Drug of choice for status epilepticus (initial)?
Lorazepam
Preferred over diazepam.

Q61. Drug causing myopathy when combined with statins?
Gemfibrozil
↑ statin levels via CYP inhibition.

Q62. Drug contraindicated with MAO inhibitors?
SSRIs
Risk of serotonin syndrome.

Q63. Drug used in cyanide poisoning apart from hydroxocobalamin?
Sodium thiosulfate
Donates sulfur to detoxify cyanide.

Q64. Drug causing orange discoloration of body fluids?
Rifampin
Harmless but alarming to patients.

Q65. Antibiotic causing tendon rupture?
Fluoroquinolones
Especially in elderly or steroid use.

Q66. Drug class causing red man syndrome?
Vancomycin
Histamine-mediated reaction.

Q67. Drug class associated with oto- and nephrotoxicity?
Aminoglycosides
Eg: gentamicin.

Q68. Drug of choice in hypertensive emergency with renal failure?
Labetalol
Safe in CKD.

Q69. Drug used in paracetamol overdose?
N-acetylcysteine
Replenishes glutathione.

Q70. Drug with "cheese reaction" when taken with tyramine foods?
MAO inhibitors
Causes hypertensive crisis.

Q71. Which drug prolongs PR interval and used in PSVT?
Adenosine
DOC for AVNRT.

Q72. Immunosuppressant that binds FKBP but inhibits mTOR?
Sirolimus
Not nephrotoxic.

Q73. Drug of choice in neuroleptic malignant syndrome?
Dantrolene or bromocriptine
Skeletal muscle relaxant.

Q74. Vitamin used to prevent isoniazid neurotoxicity?
Vitamin B6 (pyridoxine)
Prescribed with INH.

Q75. Antiemetic safe in pregnancy?
Doxylamine + pyridoxine
FDA category A.

Q76. Drug used for androgenic alopecia?
Finasteride
5-alpha reductase inhibitor.

Q77. Drug used to treat postmenopausal osteoporosis and breast cancer?
Raloxifene
SERM.

Q78. Mechanism of action of denosumab?
RANKL inhibitor
Reduces osteoclast activity.

Q79. Drug causing fanconi syndrome?
Tenofovir
Proximal tubular dysfunction.

Q80. Which SERM causes endometrial hyperplasia?
Tamoxifen
Acts as estrogen agonist on uterus.

Q81. Drug for gestational diabetes mellitus (GDM)?
Insulin
Does not cross placenta.

Q82. Monoclonal antibody against IL-6 receptor?
Tocilizumab
Used in cytokine storm, RA.

Q83. Long-acting insulin preparation?
Insulin glargine
24-hour basal control.

Q84. Drug used in pheochromocytoma before surgery?
Phenoxybenzamine
Irreversible α-blocker.

Q85. Drug causing lupus-like syndrome?
Hydralazine
Also procainamide.

Q86. Drug for chronic myeloid leukemia (CML)?
Imatinib
BCR-ABL tyrosine kinase inhibitor.

Q87. SGLT2 inhibitors reduce what apart from blood sugar?
Cardiovascular risk & proteinuria
Renoprotective.

Q88. Statin with least drug interaction risk?
Pravastatin
Not metabolized by CYP.

Q89. Anticoagulant with lowest HIT risk?
Fondaparinux
Synthetic factor Xa inhibitor.

Q90. Drug used in treatment-resistant depression (IV)?
Ketamine
NMDA receptor antagonist.

Q91. Anti-VEGF drug injected intravitreally in AMD?
Ranibizumab
Blocks neovascularization.

Q92. Hormone analog used in uterine fibroids & precocious puberty?
Leuprolide
GnRH analog.

Q93. Drug that delays labor in preterm contractions?
Nifedipine
Tocolytic.

Q94. Antiviral causing hyperbilirubinemia in neonates?
Atazanavir
Protease inhibitor.

Q95. Drug causing dry cough and angioedema?
ACE inhibitors
Due to bradykinin accumulation.

Q96. Which antibiotic causes red discoloration of urine?
Rifampin
Harmless, but tell the patient.

Q97. Drug causing neural tube defects in pregnancy?
Valproate
Avoid in first trimester.

Q98. Drug of choice for acute variceal bleed?
Octreotide
Splanchnic vasoconstriction.

Q99. Drug of choice for BPH with hypertension?
Terazosin
Alpha-1 blocker.

Q100. Which inhalational anesthetic is contraindicated in pneumothorax?
Nitrous oxide
Expands closed air spaces.

Q101. Drug of choice for Cushing's disease (medical management)?
Ketoconazole
Inhibits steroid synthesis.

Q102. Which vitamin increases iron absorption?
Vitamin C (ascorbic acid)
Reduces Fe^{3+} to Fe^{2+}.

Q103. Monoclonal antibody targeting CD20?
Rituximab
Used in B-cell lymphomas, RA.

Q104. Drug used to prevent chemotherapy-induced neutropenia?
Filgrastim
G-CSF analog.

Q105. Antihypertensive safe in pregnancy?
Labetalol
First-line in gestational hypertension.

Q106. First-line drug for alcohol withdrawal?
Benzodiazepines
Eg: chlordiazepoxide or lorazepam.

Q107. Anticoagulant used in DVT and safe in renal failure?
Unfractionated heparin
Cleared by liver.

Q108. Antiandrogen used in prostate cancer?
Flutamide
Blocks androgen receptor.

Q109. Dopamine agonist used in hyperprolactinemia?
Cabergoline
Long-acting D2 agonist.

Q110. Drug that causes disulfiram-like reaction with alcohol?
Metronidazole
Also cefoperazone, chlorpropamide.

Q111. Antiepileptic with hepatotoxicity in children under 2?
Valproate
Monitor liver function.

Q112. Drug of choice for thyrotoxic crisis?
Propylthiouracil (PTU)
Inhibits T4 to T3 conversion.

Q113. Which anti-TB drug is hepatotoxic and causes peripheral neuropathy?
Isoniazid
Add pyridoxine.

Q114. Drug causing crystalline retinopathy?
Tamoxifen
Rare visual side effect.

Q115. Glucose-lowering drug that causes weight loss?
SGLT2 inhibitors
Also cause mild diuresis.

Q116. Antimalarial causing vivid dreams and psychosis?
Mefloquine
Used in prophylaxis.

Q117. Insulin preparation used for meal-time coverage?
Insulin lispro
Rapid-acting.

Q118. Anti-hyperlipidemic that increases triglycerides?
Bile acid sequestrants (e.g., cholestyramine)
Not used in hypertriglyceridemia.

Q119. Drug used for chemoprevention in breast cancer?
Tamoxifen
Especially ER-positive tumors.

Q120. Drug causing pancreatitis and gallstones in diabetes?
GLP-1 analogs (e.g., liraglutide)
Also causes satiety.

Q121. Anticancer drug causing hemorrhagic cystitis?
Cyclophosphamide
Prevented with MESNA.

Q122. Drug used in rheumatoid arthritis targeting IL-1?
Anakinra
Less common than anti-TNF agents.

Q123. Antidiabetic drug that delays gastric emptying?
GLP-1 agonists
Eg: exenatide.

Q124. Drug used in resistant schizophrenia?
Clozapine
Risk of agranulocytosis.

Q125. Dopaminergic drug used in Parkinson's that causes compulsive behavior?
Pramipexole
Also causes sleep attacks.

Q126. Reversal agent for dabigatran?
Idarucizumab
Specific antidote.

Q127. Antiretroviral causing bone marrow suppression?
Zidovudine
Monitor Hb and WBC.

Q128. Drug that inhibits thyroid hormone release?
Iodide (Lugol's solution)
Wolff-Chaikoff effect.

Q129. Which antipsychotic causes hyperprolactinemia most?
Risperidone
D2 blockade in tuberoinfundibular tract.

Q130. Hypoglycemic with cardiovascular benefit?
Empagliflozin (SGLT2i), liraglutide (GLP-1)
Proven in trials.

Q131. Anticancer agent causing pulmonary fibrosis?
Bleomycin
Dose-limiting toxicity.

Q132. Tyrosine kinase inhibitor for renal cell carcinoma?
Sunitinib
Also for GIST.

Q133. Immunosuppressant inhibiting purine synthesis?
Azathioprine
TPMT testing needed.

Q134. Vaccine contraindicated in pregnancy?
MMR, varicella (live vaccines)
Defer till postpartum.

Q135. Anti-TB drug causing optic neuritis?
Ethambutol
Red-green color blindness.

Q136. DOC for toxoplasmosis in pregnancy?
Spiramycin
Reduces fetal transmission.

Q137. Anticonvulsant used in neuropathic pain?
Gabapentin
Binds voltage-gated Ca^{2+} channels.

Q138. Drug used for pulmonary artery hypertension targeting endothelin?
Bosentan
Endothelin receptor antagonist.

Q139. Long-acting insulin with flat profile?
Insulin degludec
Ultra-long-acting.

Q140. Anti-diabetic that increases GLP-1 levels indirectly?
DPP-4 inhibitors (e.g., sitagliptin)
Prolong GLP-1 action.

Q141. Anticancer drug causing hand-foot syndrome?
Capecitabine
5-FU prodrug.

Q142. Antibiotic with lowest risk in pregnancy?
Penicillin
Category B.

Q143. Anti-estrogen used in infertility?
Clomiphene
Induces ovulation.

Q144. Beta-blocker preferred in asthma?
Nebivolol or cardioselective like metoprolol
Use cautiously.

Q145. Immunosuppressant with high nephrotoxicity risk?
Cyclosporine
Monitor creatinine.

Q146. Anti-TNF drug for Crohn's disease?
Infliximab
Also used in RA, psoriasis.

Q147. Topical drug for actinic keratosis?
5-Fluorouracil
Also used for skin SCC.

Q148. Oral hypoglycemic with maximum weight gain?
Sulfonylureas
Eg: glimepiride.

Q149. Which antiemetic is contraindicated in Parkinson's?
Metoclopramide
Causes extrapyramidal symptoms.

Q150. Drug used in acute intermittent porphyria?
Hemin
Downregulates ALA synthase.

Q151. Antiplatelet agent used in stroke prevention that causes neutropenia?
Ticlopidine
Rare but serious side effect.

Q152. Drug of choice for carcinoid syndrome diarrhea?
Octreotide
Somatostatin analog.

Q153. Which antidiabetic drug causes vitamin B12 deficiency?
Metformin
With long-term use.

Q154. Drug used to prevent kidney transplant rejection and gout?
Mycophenolate mofetil
Inhibits inosine monophosphate dehydrogenase.

Q155. Which antiarrhythmic causes thyroid dysfunction?
Amiodarone
Contains iodine.

Q156. Drug causing optic neuritis in TB treatment?
Ethambutol
Dose-dependent.

Q157. Agent causing SJS (Stevens-Johnson Syndrome)?
Lamotrigine
Also sulfa drugs, allopurinol.

Q158. Anticancer agent causing hemorrhagic cystitis?
Ifosfamide
Prevented by MESNA.

Q159. Which monoclonal antibody blocks PD-1?
Nivolumab
Immune checkpoint inhibitor.

Q160. Drug of choice for methemoglobinemia?
Methylene blue
Converts Fe^{3+} to Fe^{2+}.

Q161. Prokinetic drug causing Parkinsonism?
Metoclopramide
Blocks D2 receptors.

Q162. Which anti-TB drug causes psychosis?
Cycloserine
Neuropsychiatric side effects.

Q163. DOC for hydatid disease?
Albendazole
Antiparasitic.

Q164. Drug causing dry mouth, blurred vision, and tachycardia?
Atropine
Anticholinergic toxicity.

Q165. Drug-induced lupus with positive anti-histone antibodies?
Hydralazine, INH
Classically associated.

Q166. Drug used for prevention of cisplatin-induced nephrotoxicity?
Amifostine
Cytoprotective agent.

Q167. Antidiabetic that should be avoided in liver failure?
Pioglitazone
Risk of hepatotoxicity.

Q168. Antipsychotic least likely to cause extrapyramidal side effects?
Clozapine
But causes agranulocytosis.

Q169. Anti-TNF-α drug used in ulcerative colitis?
Adalimumab
Also in Crohn's and RA.

Q170. Drug used in Parkinsonism that also treats influenza A?
Amantadine
Dopamine agonist + antiviral.

Q171. Antiviral causing crystal-induced nephropathy?
Acyclovir
Maintain hydration.

Q172. Which antineoplastic causes cardiomyopathy?
Doxorubicin
Prevented with dexrazoxane.

Q173. Agent used to reverse opioid-induced constipation?
Methylnaltrexone
Peripheral μ antagonist.

Q174. Drug causing photosensitivity?
Doxycycline
Others: sulfa drugs, amiodarone.

Q175. Drug of choice for thyroid storm?
Propylthiouracil (PTU)
Blocks T4 to T3 conversion.

Q176. Antimalarial safe in pregnancy?
Chloroquine
Preferred in all trimesters.

Q177. Monoclonal antibody causing reactivation of TB?
Infliximab
Screen before initiation.

Q178. Drug causing visual halo and arrhythmia in overdose?
Digoxin
Requires Digibind.

Q179. Hypoglycemic causing megaloblastic anemia?
Metformin (rare), more often with phenytoin
Monitor B12.

Q180. Drug used for ALS (amyotrophic lateral sclerosis)?
Riluzole
Delays need for ventilation.

Q181. First-line for ectopic pregnancy?
Methotrexate
Single-dose protocol.

Q182. Drug that inhibits dihydroorotate dehydrogenase in RA?
Leflunomide
Inhibits pyrimidine synthesis.

Q183. Which AED is enzyme inducer?
Phenytoin
↑ metabolism of other drugs.

Q184. Drug of choice for post-exposure HIV prophylaxis?
Tenofovir + lamivudine + dolutegravir
Within 72 hours.

Q185. Reversal agent for rivaroxaban (factor Xa inhibitor)?
Andexanet alfa
Specific antidote.

Q186. Drug causing galactorrhea due to dopamine blockade?
Antipsychotics (especially risperidone)
D2 antagonism.

Q187. Immunosuppressant that inhibits purine synthesis via IMPDH?
Mycophenolate mofetil
Acts on lymphocytes.

Q188. Drug used to prevent neural tube defect in pregnancy?
Folic acid
Start preconceptionally.

Q189. Anticonvulsant safe in pregnancy?
Levetiracetam
Minimal teratogenicity.

Q190. Antifungal causing gynecomastia in long-term use?
Ketoconazole
Anti-androgenic effect.

Q191. DOC for febrile neutropenia?
Cefepime or piperacillin-tazobactam
Broad-spectrum coverage.

Q192. Topical agent for tinea corporis?
Clotrimazole
Azole antifungal.

Q193. Antiepileptic causing weight gain and tremor?
Valproate
Also hepatotoxic.

Q194. Antiviral safe in pregnancy for herpes?
Acyclovir
Used in recurrent genital HSV.

Q195. Drug used to treat refractory ascites in cirrhosis?
Midodrine + albumin + diuretics
Improves renal perfusion.

Q196. Drug causing sexual dysfunction in males with BPH?
Finasteride
5α-reductase inhibitor.

Q197. DOC for hepatic encephalopathy?
Lactulose
Traps ammonia in colon.

Q198. Antibiotic with concentration-dependent killing?
Aminoglycosides
Once-daily dosing.

Q199. Antiplatelet safe for aspirin-allergic patients?
Clopidogrel
ADP receptor blocker.

Q200. First-line therapy for diabetic gastroparesis?
Metoclopramide
Prokinetic + antiemetic.

www.ingramcontent.com/pod-product-compliance
Ingram Content Group UK Ltd.
Pitfield, Milton Keynes, MK11 3LW, UK
UKHW061539190726
13845UKWH00031B/1119

9 789334 29198